COLOUR GUIDE

PICTURE TESTS

Orthopaedics and Trauma

R. L. Huckstep CMG FTS Hon MD (NSW)
MA MD (Cantab) FRCS (Eng) FRCS (Ed) FRACS FA.Orth.A.

Emeritus Professor of Traumatic and Orthopaedic Surgery, University of New South Wales and Consultant Orthopaedic Surgeon, Prince of Wales Hospital, Sydney, Australia; *Formerly* Foundation Professor and Head, Department of Traumatic and Orthopaedic Surgery, and Chairman, School of Surgery, University of New South Wales; Vice-President, Australian Orthopaedic Association; Professor of Orthopaedic Surgery, Makerere University, Kampala, Uganda; Hunterian Professor, Royal College of Surgeons of England; Corresponding Editor, Journal of Bone and Joint Surgery, Injury and the Archives of Orthopaedic and Traumatic Surgery

Eugene Sherry MB ChB (Otago) MPH (Sydney) MD (NSW)
FRACS (Orth)

Orthopaedic Surgeon, Hills Private Hospital, Sydney; *Formerly* Director, Ski Injury Clinic, Perisher Valley, New South Wales, Australia

D0217626

Churchill Livingstone

EDINBURGH LONDON MADRID MELBOURNE NEW YORK TOKYO 1994

Preface

This quiz atlas on orthopaedics and trauma has been written as a simple revision text, and includes colour prints and X-rays of both common and unusual injuries and orthopaedic conditions. The illustrations are based on the authors' teaching over many years of medical students, doctors, nurses and paramedical staff. Most of the cases in this quiz were the senior author's own patients. The questions have been designed to be brief and to the point, whilst the answers have sometimes been enlarged to include a differential diagnosis and treatment, where relevant.

The book has also been designed to be complementary to the senior author's two books *A Simple Guide to Trauma* and *A Simple Guide to Orthopaedics*. These two books, plus the bibliography of other recommended books, should enable the reader to obtain further information on both diagnosis and treatment, if required.

It is hoped that these picture tests will prove of particular value to senior medical students and junior doctors, as well as to surgical registrars and residents in training. It could also be of value to general practitioners, as well as to doctors, nurses, physiotherapists and paramedical personnel working in orthopaedic outpatient departments and accident and emergency centres.

We should like particularly to thank Bruce Cooper, Louise Delaney Angela Georgopoulos, Graeme Hall, Antony Henderson, Michael Huckstep, Michael Maley and particularly Ralph Mobbs for their help in editing the questions and with the collection of the photographs and X-rays.

We are also grateful to Mr. Alex Benjamin, FRCS, for providing several excellent illustrations and X-rays, and to Professor E. H. Bates for Figures 24 and 39. We should also like to thank Julian Ayer, Renee Hannan, Michael Hunter, Mark Jackson, Phillip Lutton, Michelle Miller and Carl O'Kane for their help.

We are indebted to the late Dr. Hugh Smith, through whose generosity the Orthopaedic Research Department of the University of New South Wales was established, and to Mr. Ronald Wright for his help through the University of New South Wales Foundation.

We would like to thank the staff of the University of New South Wales Medical Illustration Department at the Prince of Wales Hospital, Sydney, and in particular, Mr. Michael Oakey and Mr. Donald Strachan, for their help with the photography of the X-rays and of some of the patients. The staff of Churchill Livingstone, and in particular, Mr. Jim Killgore, have been, as usual, most helpful in the publication of this book.

Sydney   R. L. H.
1994   E. S.

Contents

Orthopaedics—Questions

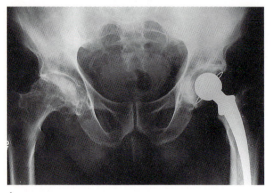

1.

a. List some common indications for a total hip replacement.
b. What are the X-ray features shown on the right hip?
c. What are the likely clinical history and signs in this patient?
d. List the types of treatment available in osteoarthritis.

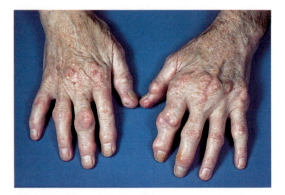

2. **A middle-aged female presents with painful deformities of both hands.**

a. What is the deformity? Comment on the disease process.
b. Discuss the possible treatment.

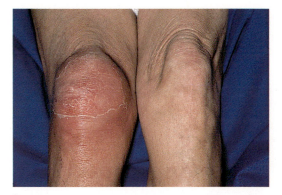

3. A 60-year-old male plumber with anterior right knee pain.

a. What is the diagnosis?
b. What patients develop this problem?
c. What treatment can be proposed?

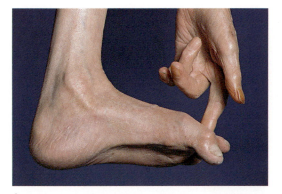

4. It was not possible to extend passively or actively the 3rd, 4th and 5th digits of the hands and feet of this middle-aged male.

a. What is the diagnosis? Name the anatomical structure involved.
b. What treatment can be offered?
c. List several associated medical conditions.

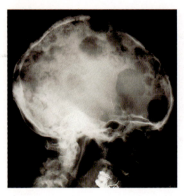

5. A 68-year-old man with severe low back pain. An X-ray of his skull is shown.

a What is the diagnosis?
b. What other tests are required to make a diagnosis?
c. How would you treat this patient?

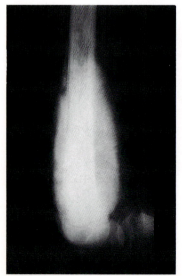

6. A 15-year-old boy with increasing pain and swelling of his lower thigh. There is a history of a fall 2 months ago. Aspiration of the swelling revealed a large collection of sterile pus.

a. What are the X-ray features shown?
b. What is the most likely diagnosis?
c. How would you investigate and manage this patient?

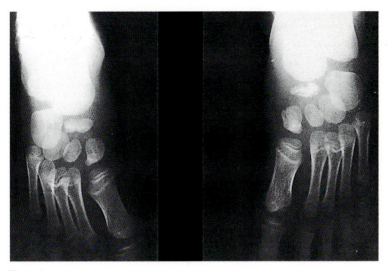

7.

a. What condition is causing the mid-foot deformity of this child?
b. What are the physical signs?

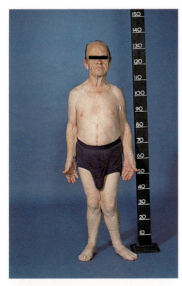

8. A dwarf who was severely mentally handicapped until the age of 48. Following treatment with hormones he was able to look after himself and was intellectually much improved.

a. What is the diagnosis?
b. What are the orthopaedic manifestations of this condition?

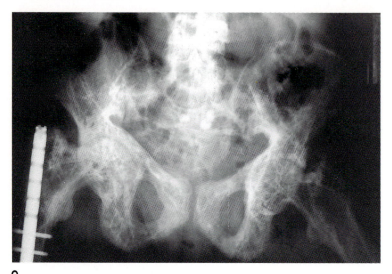

9. X-rays of a patient with a painful right hip.

a. What is the diagnosis?
b. List the clinical features and associated complications.

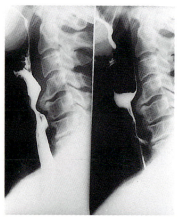

10.

a. What investigation is being shown here?
b. What symptom may the patient have been complaining of?
c. Discuss the diagnosis.

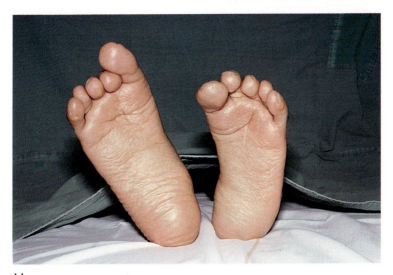

11. What could account for the different foot sizes?

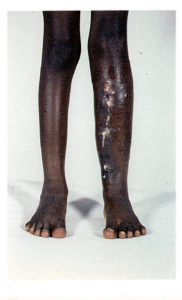

12. Deep-seated pain in the lower leg of a 14-year-old boy injured 2 years ago.

a. Discuss the differential diagnosis.
b. Outline the treatment.

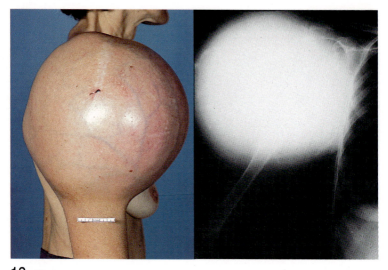

13. This 70-year-old female presented with a bony swelling of the shoulder girdle increasing in size over 6 months.

a. What is the most likely diagnosis in an elderly lady?
b. What is the differential diagnosis?

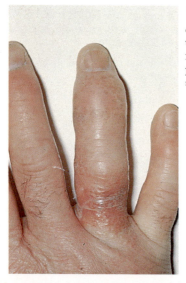

14. Given the history of sudden onset in bed at 3 am, what is the likely diagnosis in these fingers which had had five previous episodes of a sudden swelling?

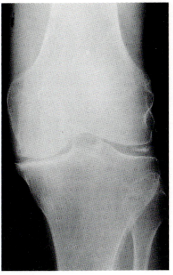

15. **An elderly female with a painful knee.**

a. What is the pathognomonic feature on the X-ray?
b. What is the diagnosis?
c. Discuss the likely causes.
d. What is the treatment?

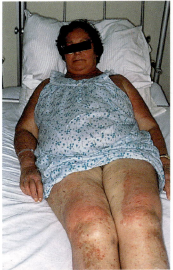

16. **A middle-aged woman with a flare up of her skin condition, associated with painful hands and feet.**

a. What is the diagnosis?
b. Name a complication of this disease pertaining to the spine.
c. Is there a genetic marker for this disease?
d. List the various drug treatments to combat the joint symptoms.

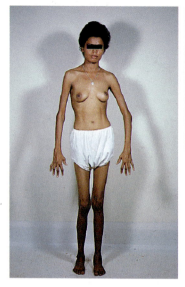

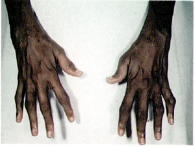

17. A young female with painful joints of several months' duration.

a. Discuss the diagnosis.
b. What clinical features are demonstrated?
c. List some non-articular signs of this disease.
d. List three complications which may occur.

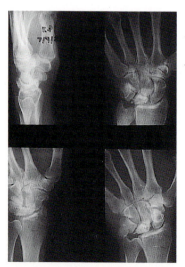

18. A 40-year-old male complains of a painful wrist.

a. Describe the X-ray appearances.
b. Discuss the diagnosis.

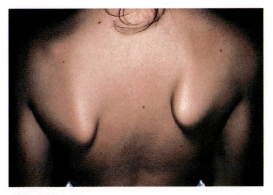

19.

a. What is this young girl's problem?
b. What would be a differential diagnosis?

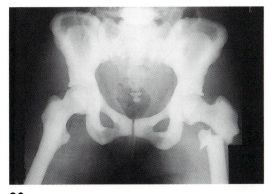

20. The X-ray shows a three part subtrochanteric fracture of the femur with marked displacement and angulation following minimal trauma.

a. What is the underlying condition and its types?
b. What is the treatment?

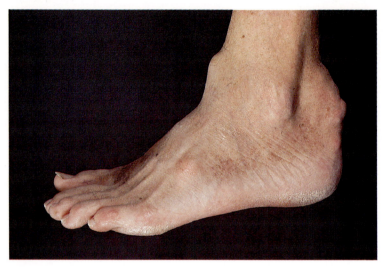

21.

a. What is the differential diagnosis of lumps such as these over the back of the calcaneus?

b. How may a diagnosis be confirmed?

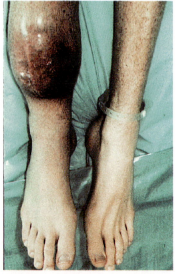

22.

a. What is the differential diagnosis of an increasing swelling over the mid-shaft of the tibia of several months' duration in a 16-year-old boy? Aspiration revealed sterile pus despite no previous antibiotics and no sinus.

b. What should be done for the patient?

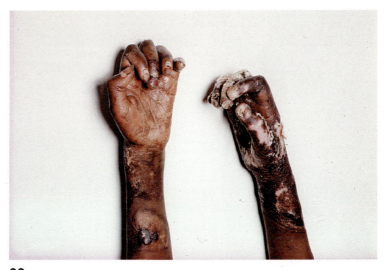

23. **A young African is seen with deformed hypopigmented and anaesthetic hands.**

a. What is the most likely diagnosis?
b. How would this patient be treated?

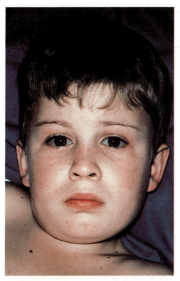

24.

a. What is the diagnosis?
b. What are the characteristic features of this condition and likely prognosis?

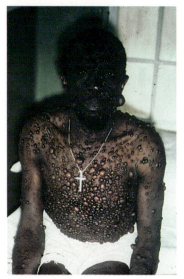

25.

a. What is the diagnosis?
b. What are the clinical manifestations and possible sequelae?

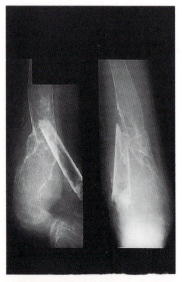

26.

a. What condition is shown here?
b. What are the typical X-ray features?
c. List three complications.

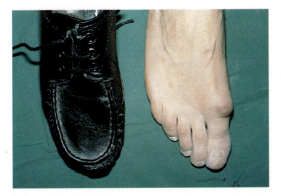

27. **A 55-year-old man with slight pain of several years'
duration in the great toe on walking.**

a. What is the most likely diagnosis?
b. Why can the diagnosis be made even before the patient removes
his shoe?

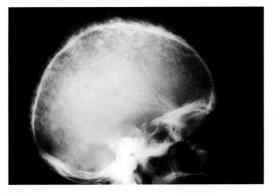

28.

a. Describe the appearance of this skull.
b. What is the diagnosis?

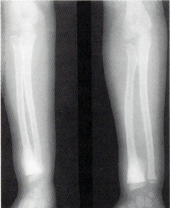

(a)

29. A 7-year-old boy is brought to hospital with a slightly tender right wrist with a slowly growing swelling on the front of the radius (a). This has required a below elbow amputation. Several months later an X-ray of his amputation stump showed various sclerotic opacities (b), as did his chest X-ray (c) and several of his other bones. What is the likely diagnosis?

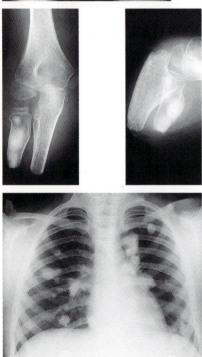

(b)

(c)

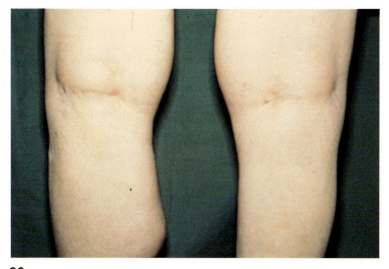

30. **A 60-year-old female complains of a painless swelling behind her left knee which appears to have increased in size over the last few months.**

a. What is the most likely diagnosis and cause?
b. What would be the most effective treatment?

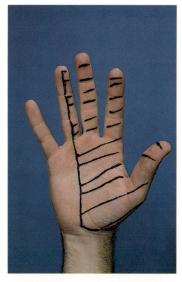

31. **This patient complained of pain and paraesthesia in the distribution as shown.**

a. Name the nerve that supplies this region.
b. If the patient is awoken at night by the pain and derives relief by shaking the hand, what is the likely diagnosis?
c. Discuss the treatment for this common condition.

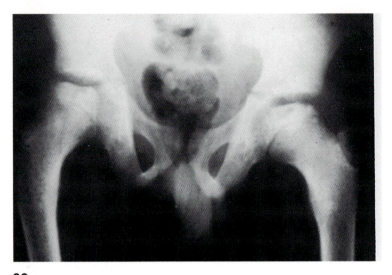

32. The X-ray of a 7-year-old boy with an intermittent limp and ache of his hips.

a. What is the likely diagnosis?
b. What are the symptoms and signs?
c. What is the treatment?

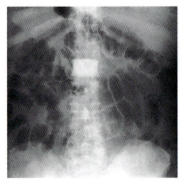

33. An elderly man with known prostate cancer.

a. Describe the X-ray.
b. List the other primary sites that could give you this appearance.

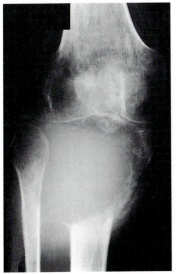

34.
a. What is the diagnosis of this painful lesion in a 35-year-old female?
b. What is the pathognomonic feature of this lesion?
c. List the complications.
d. Discuss the treatment.

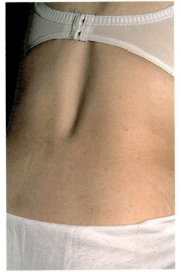

35. A 25-year-old female complains of vague lower back pain of several years' duration. She is otherwise well.

a. What is the diagnosis?
b. What is the likely cause?
c. What is the usual site of this deformity?

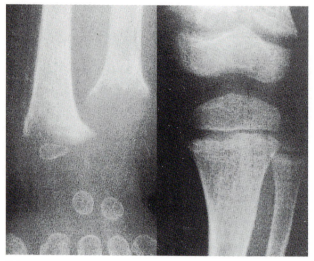

36.

a. What radiological features are seen on this X-ray?
b. What is the disease?

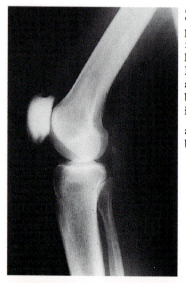

37. A 70-year-old male has had pain over his right knee cap for 5 years. He feels that it is also larger than the opposite patella. His left tibia and left femur have also been slightly tender and bent over the past few years. He is otherwise well.

a. Describe the X-ray appearance.
b. Discuss the most likely diagnosis.

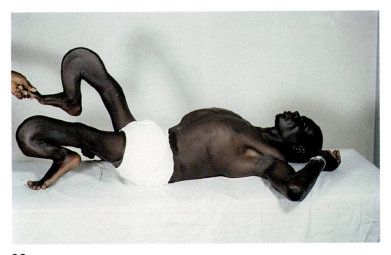

38. A financially successful, uneducated beggar in an African country.

a. What deformity does this man have?
b. What is the most likely cause?
c. What would be his best treatment in a poor African country?

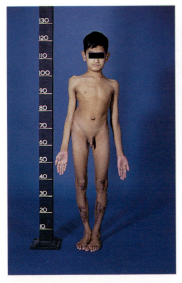

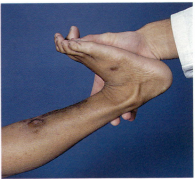

39.

a. What syndrome does this boy have?
b. What are the characteristic features of this syndrome?

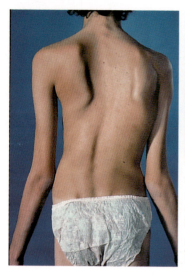

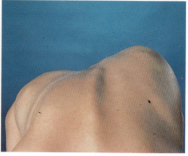

40. **An adolescent girl with a spinal deformity which is more obvious when she bends forward.**

a. What is the diagnosis?
b. What is the treatment?

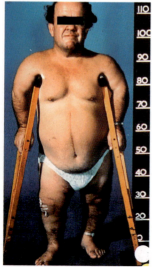

41.

a. What is the diagnosis?
b. What is the mode of inheritance?
c. What are the characteristic features of this condition?

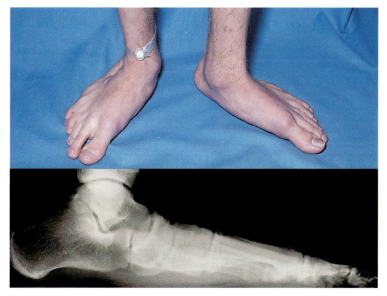

42.

a. Name this condition.
b. What are the causes?
c. What is the treatment?

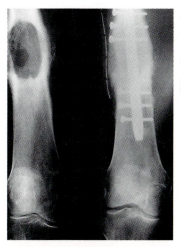

43. A slightly tender lesion of the right thigh with no history of trauma or infection in a 65-year-old woman.

a. What is the most likely diagnosis?
b. How is it best treated?

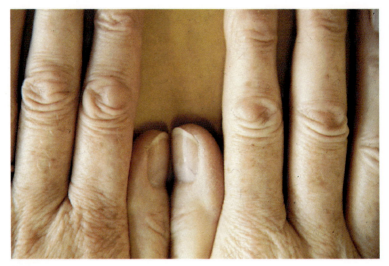

44.

a. What interesting sign can be seen in this picture?
b. Name the condition of which this is diagnostic.

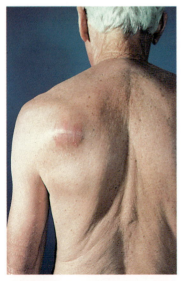

45. **An elderly man who is
otherwise well with a 6-month
history of a painless bony
swelling increasing in size over
his scapula. There is no history
of trauma.**

a. What is the most likely
   diagnosis?
b. What is the scar likely to be?
c. Discuss the treatment and
   prognosis.

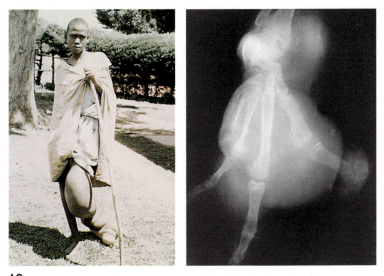

46. **An African patient presents with this deformity.**

a. Name the most likely diagnosis.
b. What is the differential diagnosis?
c. Is treatment necessary here?

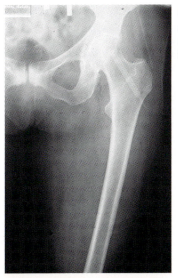

47. **An interesting hip X-ray of a healthy woman. Describe the abnormality seen in the left hip in this X-ray.**

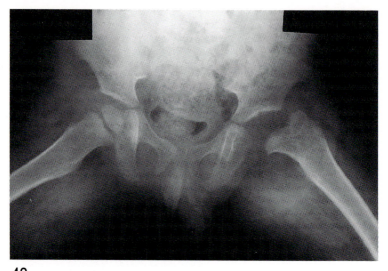

48. **A child with a limp and a hypermobile painless hip.**

a. What is the most likely diagnosis?
b. Discuss the initial management of this patient in the early stage.

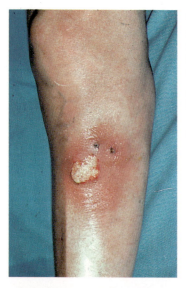

49. **A middle-aged overweight male with a painful area of 3 months' duration over his upper tibia, which was initially chalk white in colour.**

a. What is the diagnosis?
b. Which other area is usually involved?
c. How would you treat this condition?

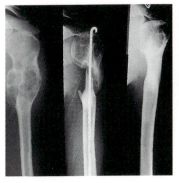

50. **The X-rays of the left humerus of a nurse aged 18 with recent pain and swelling of her arm.**

a. What is the likely diagnosis?
b. What is a likely complication?
c. Describe the treatment.

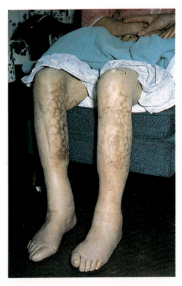

51. **A 75-year-old woman who lives in Scotland. She presents with discoloration of the outer side of the left calf and inner aspect of the right leg. What is the diagnosis?**

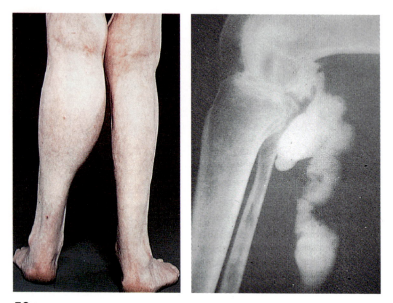

52. A middle-aged patient with osteoarthritis of the knees presents with sudden onset of right calf pain.

a. What is the diagnosis?
b. How can it be confirmed?
c. What is the treatment?

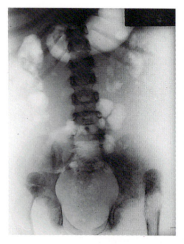

53. A 4-year-old boy who was quite normal until one month previously. He then, for no apparent reason, became febrile and complained of severe pain in both groins. He has remained febrile and ill, and has been unable to walk since then.

a. Describe the X-ray.
b. What is the diagnosis, and why?

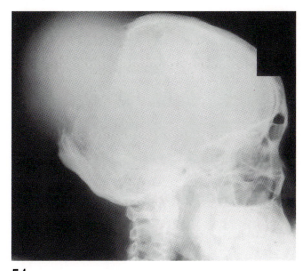

54. A 60-year-old female in Africa treated by the village 'doctor' for 3 years for a slowly growing swelling over the back of her head. She has a slight headache, is unsteady on her feet, but is otherwise well. What is the likely diagnosis?

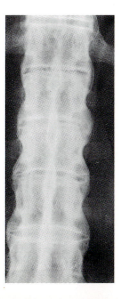

55.

a. Describe the X-ray, and the most likely diagnosis.
b. Discuss some systemic complications of this disease.

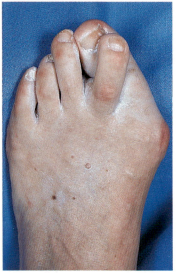

56.

a. Name this condition.
b. What is the treatment?

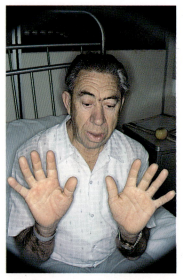

57.

a. What condition does this man have?
b. What are the associated orthopaedic problems?

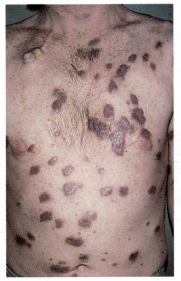

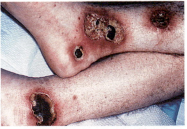

58. A 35-year-old male who has not been feeling well recently.

a. What disease does he have?
b. What are the orthopaedic manifestations of this condition?

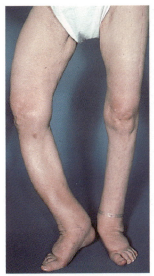

59. Anterolateral bowing of the tibia and femur.

a. What is the most likely diagnosis?
b. What symptoms could this produce?
c. Discuss your treatment.

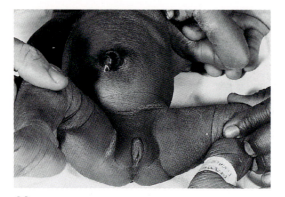

60. **An African neonate with limited abduction of the right hip.**

a. What is the most likely diagnosis, and is this common in children?
b. What are the predisposing factors?
c. How would you treat this?

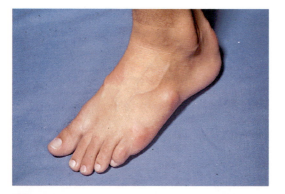

61. **A young boy from Bondi in Sydney presents with slightly tender lumps overlying the bases of both his fifth metatarsals. He is a keen surfer.**

a. What is the diagnosis?
b. What is the treatment?

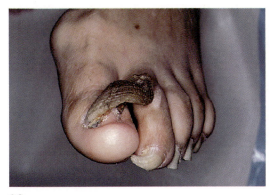

62.

a. Name this deformity.
b. What is the treatment?

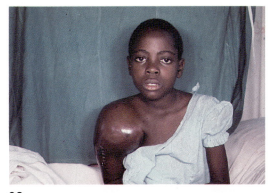

63. A teenage girl with a massive painful swelling of the shoulder girdle, increasing over a period of only six months.

a. What is the likely diagnosis?
b. What investigations should be performed?
c. What is the treatment?

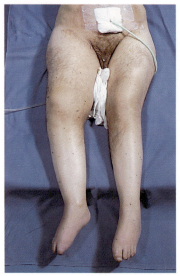

64. A man aged 50 with a congenital defect of his lower spine.

a. What is this man's condition?
b. Name some features illustrated of this disease.
c. What are some other associated characteristics of this condition?

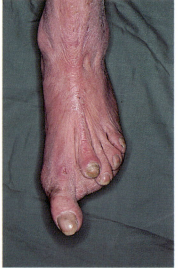

65.

a. What is the diagnosis in this foot?
b. How should it be treated?

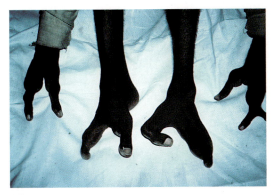

66.

a. What is the diagnosis?
b. Is treatment necessary in this case?

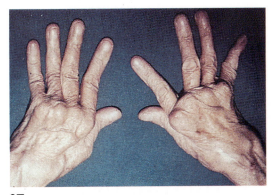

67. These are the hands of a middle-aged female.

a. State the diagnosis and discuss her disorder.
b. Name the deformity of the left thumb and its significance.

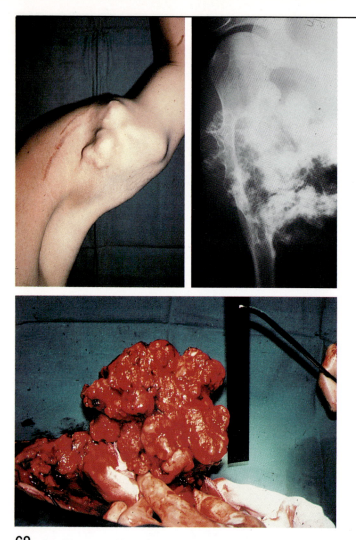

68. An 18-year-old male presented with a painful irregular large bony lump on his left upper arm which was increasing in size and causing vascular and neurological compression and paralysis of his left arm and hand. There were similar small bony lumps on other parts of his body but they were asymptomatic.

a. What is the likely diagnosis?
b. What other bones are likely to be involved?
c. Does it require treatment?

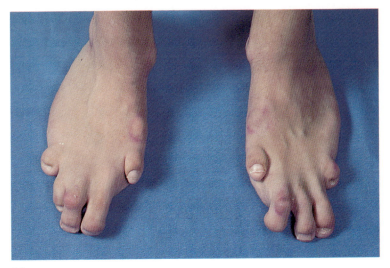

69.

a. What deformity does this patient have?
b. Name the associated functional deficiency.
c. Discuss what treatment would be required.

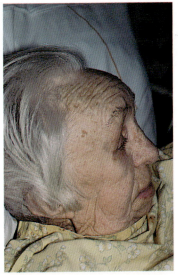

70.

a. What condition does this female have?
b. What symptoms may the patient experience?

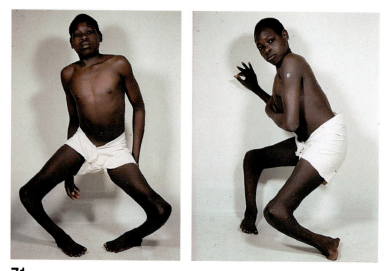

71. A teenager with increasing deformity of both knees since birth.

a. Name the deformity.
b. Give the eponym given to this condition.
c. How should this be treated?

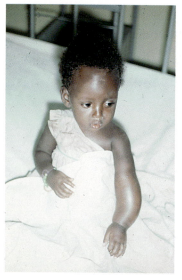

72. A young child presents with severe pain and a tense swelling of the forearm of 5 days' duration. There is no history of trauma.

a. Give the two most likely diagnoses.
b. List the investigations which would be useful.

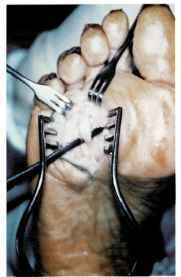

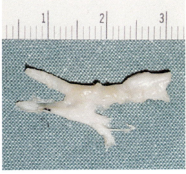

73. A specimen excised from a patient's painful forefoot.

a. What is this mass?
b. What is the differential diagnosis?
c. Discuss the treatment.

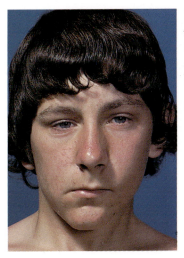

74. A 14-year-old male with a neck problem for many years and recent eye problems.

a. What is the likely diagnosis?
b. What is the treatment at this stage?
c. What is the differential diagnosis of neck deformities?

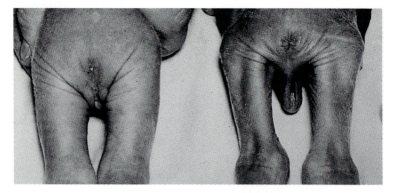

75. A pair of twins—a boy and a girl. The mother complained that the boy's hips 'click' when she changes his nappies.

a. What is the diagnosis?
b. Is this condition more common in boys or girls?

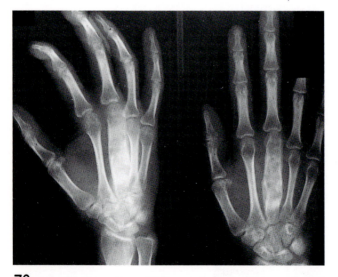

76. The X-rays of a middle-aged male who presented with a painless bony swelling of his hand increasing in size over several months.

a. What is the differential diagnosis?
b. What is the treatment?

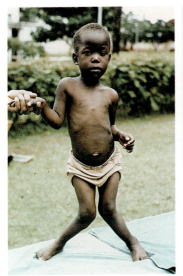

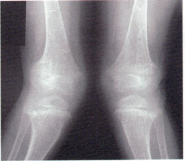

77.

a. What is the diagnosis?
b. What are the causes?
c. What is the treatment?

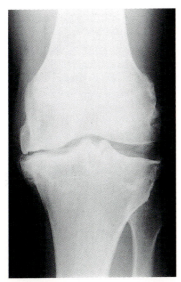

78.

a. What disease does this patient have?
b. What signs and symptoms would be expected?
c. How can it be treated?

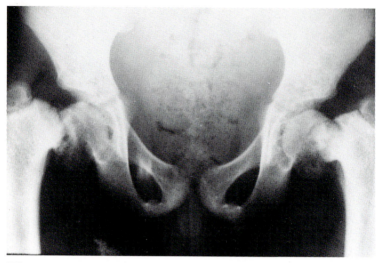

79.

a. Name this hip condition.
b. What are the likely causes?
c. What is the likely sequel to this deformity?

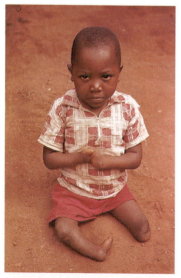

80. A 5-year-old boy presented like this with no scars.

a. What deformities does the boy have and their cause?
b. How can he be treated?

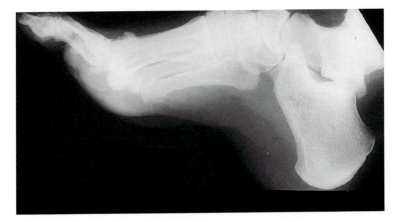

81.

a. What is the condition depicted here?
b. With what condition is this associated?

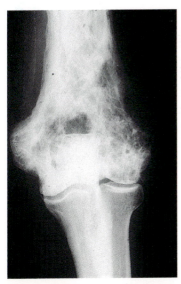

82. A 70-year-old male complains of increasing pain in his elbow.

a. What is the underlying diagnosis?
b. Which complication has developed?
c. What is the likely prognosis?

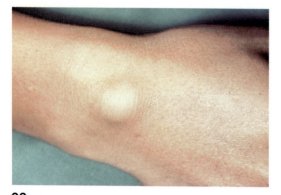

83. **This picture shows a painless firm swelling over the dorsum of a wrist.**

a. What mass is being demonstrated here?
b. What is the histology of the mass?
c. How would it be treated?

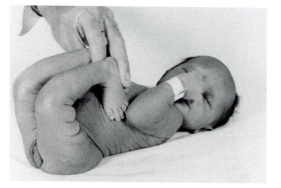

84.

a. What deformity is being demonstrated here?
b. How would you treat this patient?

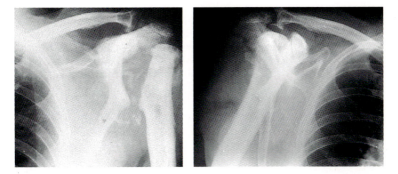

85. The X-rays of a 54-year-old man presenting with a painless swelling of both his shoulders with an increased range of all shoulder movements. There is no history of trauma or infection.

a. Name the likely diagnosis.
b. What other clinical features might you expect?
c. What is the most likely cause?

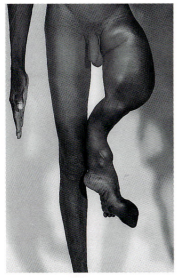

86.

a. What deformities are depicted here in this long-standing deformed right leg in a 25-year-old male with a recent slightly tender enlargement of the big toe?
b. What is the most likely diagnosis?
c. What is the best treatment?

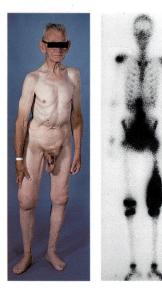

87. A 70-year-old male with Paget's disease with a 4-month swelling of his lower right thigh. A bone scan was carried out and is shown.

a. What is the most likely diagnosis and differential diagnosis?
b. Discuss the treatment and prognosis.

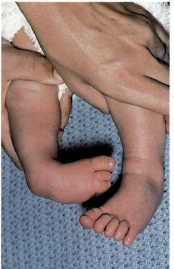

88.

a. What is this child's condition?
b. What is a possible associated deficiency?
c. Discuss the treatment.

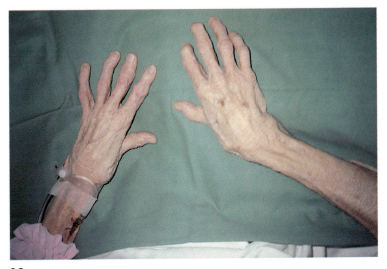

89. The hands of an elderly female who was admitted to hospital for a hip replacement.

a. What is the diagnosis?
b. Discuss the disease and the radiological findings.
c. Name the swellings over the distal interphalangeal joints.

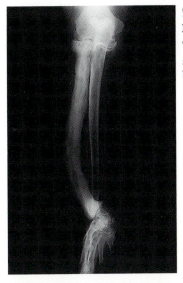

90. A warm slightly tender lesion in the radius with bony overgrowth and bowing.

a. Give the diagnosis.
b. What tests may help confirm the diagnosis?

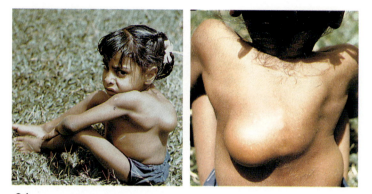

91. An African child with a spinal deformity.

a. What is the most likely cause?
b. Name this deformity.
c. What are the possible complications?

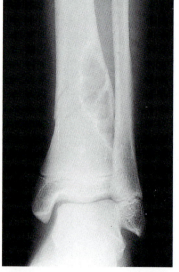

92.

a. What is the diagnosis?
b. Discuss the treatment.

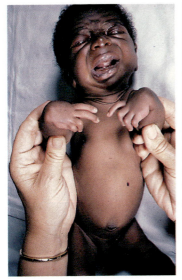

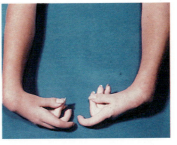

93. **An African baby and an adult, both born with hand and wrist deformities.**

a. Describe the deformity.
b. Name the syndrome and give the likely cause?

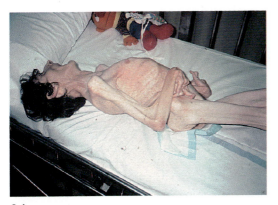

94. **A 53-year-old female who has been in institutional care all her life.**

a. Describe the deformities of this woman.
b. What is the most likely diagnosis?
c. What other orthopaedic problems do such patients have?

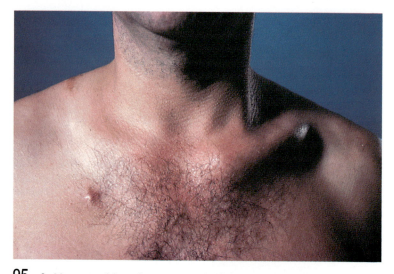

95. **A 32-year-old male presented with extreme bone tenderness over his inner clavicle.**

a. What is the diagnosis?
b. Discuss the investigations and treatment.

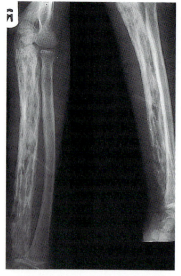

96. **This patient, from a tropical region of Australia, presented with chronic pain and swelling of the forearm. The patient had been unwell with fever, malaise and chills.**

a. What is the diagnosis?
b. What other sites may be involved?
c. Which groups of patients are particularly susceptible?

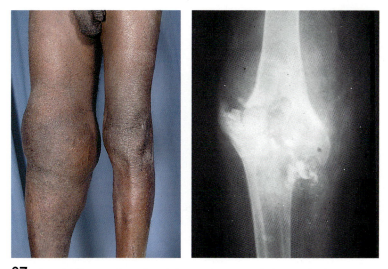

97. **A middle-aged male with an almost painless tubular swelling of an unstable knee.**

a. What is the most likely diagnosis?
b. What are the causes of relatively painless mobile joints with cartilage and bone destruction?

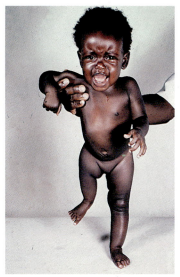

98.

a. What is the cause of the deformity of this child's right leg?
b. Discuss the possible aetiological factors.
c. What are the associated features?

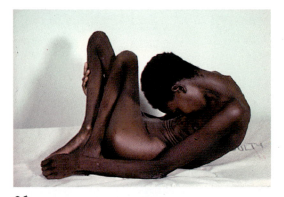

99. **An 18-year-old African female with a 3-year history of progressive deformity. Her sister died of a similar condition.**

a. Describe her neck and hip postures.
b. What is the most likely cause?
c. What is the treatment?

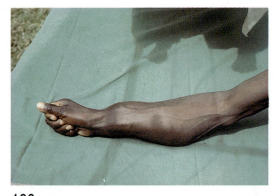

100. **This middle-aged male presented with two painless, very firm swellings over his right forearm attached to the ulna and increasing in size over two years. What is the differential diagnosis?**

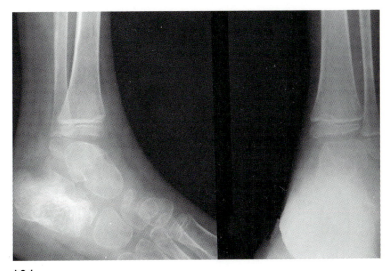

101. A painful heel in a child.

a. What is the diagnosis?
b. Describe the mechanism.
c. Outline your plan of management.

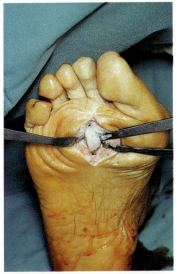

102.

a. The third metatarsal head is being excised for pain in an elderly woman. Why has this lump become painful?
b. Who is likely to have this problem, and how is it treated?

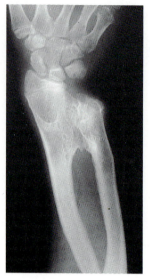

103.

a. Name this condition.
b. What is the resulting deformity?
c. What is the treatment?

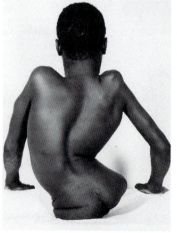

104.

a Name the deformity depicted here.
b. What is its most likely cause?

Trauma—Questions

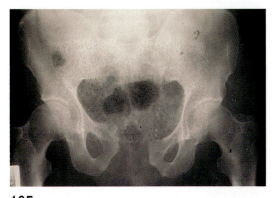

105. **This unfortunate lady was run over by a small car.**

a. Describe this X-ray and give a diagnosis in light of the history.
b. Discuss the basis of treatment in this patient.
c. List the common complications and one painful, disabling late complication.

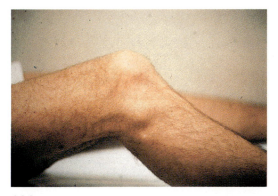

106. **A young male with a past history of injury to his knee.**

a. What is the likely diagnosis of this firm swelling on the lateral side of the knee?
b. Describe the nature of the swelling on palpation.

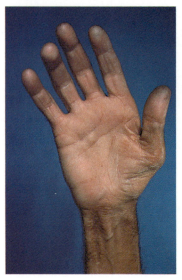

107. **This 52-year-old male presented several months after an injury to his wrist.**

a. Which nerve has been compromised?
b. Describe the associated sensory loss present.
c. How may this injury occur?

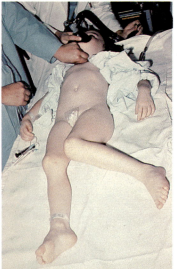

108.

a. What is the diagnosis and the deformity?
b. Describe the method of treatment.
c. List four important complications.

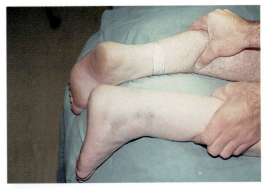

109.

a. What is the diagnosis? Name the test being performed.
b. What movement would be affected?
c. Outline the treatment regime.

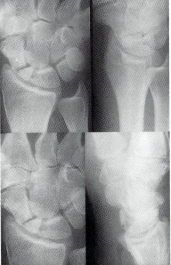

110.

a. What is the diagnosis?
b. Discuss the treatment.
c. Enumerate the main complications.

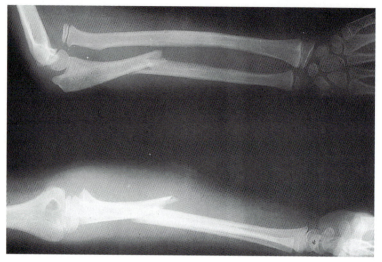

111.

a. Name and describe this injury.
b. How would you treat this injury in a child?
c. List the main complications of this injury.

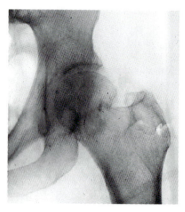

112. This elderly lady had a fall down several stairs. She presented in pain with the left leg shortened, externally rotated and adducted.

a. Discuss a simple classification for injuries of the hip.
b. What complication may occur if this injury is left untreated?
c. Would a hip replacement be a reasonable treatment regime for this patient?

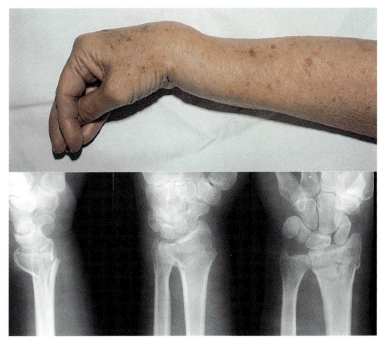

113.

a. What is the diagnosis and X-ray features?
b. How would you treat this patient?
c. What complications may this patient develop?

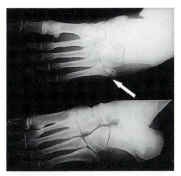

114. A lunch-time jogger presents with a painful left foot.

a. Describe the injury. What other structures may be injured?
b. Describe the mechanism of injury.
c. Comment on the possible treatment. Discuss the prognosis.

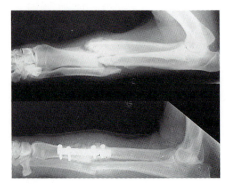

115.

a. What is the diagnosis?
b. What is the treatment?

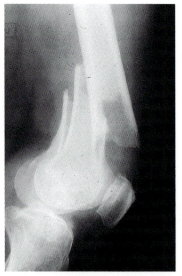

116.

a. What is the diagnosis? List six possible complications.
b. What is the standard treatment?
c. Why are these injuries especially a problem in children?

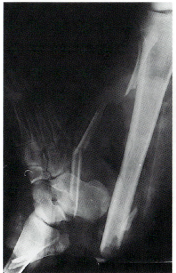

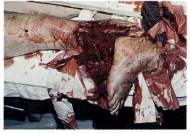

117.

a. What is the diagnosis?
b. Outline your emergency treatment.
c. What short- and long-term complications may develop?

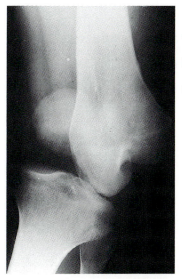

118.

a. What has happened with this man's knee?
b. List the structures which may have been damaged.
c. After your initial assessment of the patient, what is your plan of action?

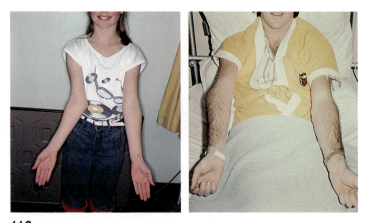

119. **A young girl (left) presents with a deformity of the elbow.**

a. What is the most common cause, or what is the cause?
b. What is a late complication of this condition and how can it be treated?
c. Name the elbow deformity in the man (right) and its most likely cause.

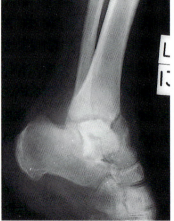

120.

a. What is the diagnosis?
b. Name the major complication.
c. Briefly discuss the treatment.

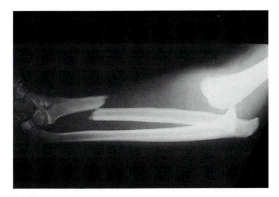

121. **This injury was sustained after a severe fall on the hand from a height.**

a. Describe the injuries in this X-ray.
b. Name the nerves possibly injured here.

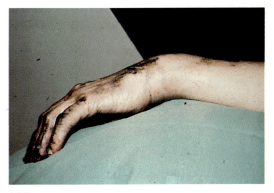

122.

a. What is the diagnosis?
b. Describe the initial management.
c. Discuss the complications.

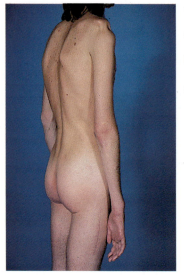

123.

a. List the features seen and discuss the differential diagnosis.
b. Give two common traumatic causes for this condition.
c. What deformity will develop over time with this injury? How can it be prevented?

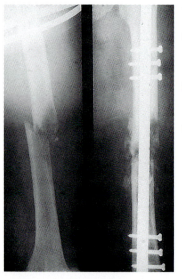

124.

a. Describe the fracture in a middle-aged woman which occurred when she was walking up stairs.
b. What aetiological factors should be considered with this fracture following minimal trauma?
c. Discuss the treatment.

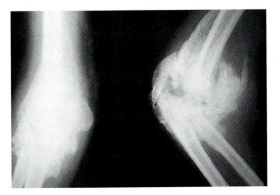

125.

a. Name the condition seen in this elbow.
b. List some other sites affected.
c. How has this condition arisen?

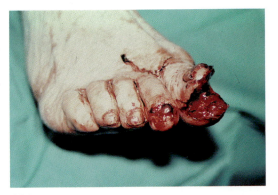

126. This 28-year-old man had an unfortunate accident in his garden.

a. Describe the injury and the cause.
b. What is the first aid management?
c. What are the likely complications?

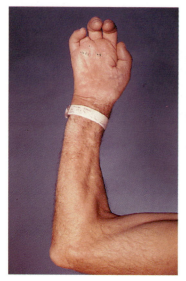

127. **A young male with a severely comminuted fracture of the radius and ulna several months ago now presents with complications.**

a. Name this condition and describe the deformities seen.
b. What structures have been compromised?
c. List the symptoms and signs of ischaemia in the forearm following a severe fracture.

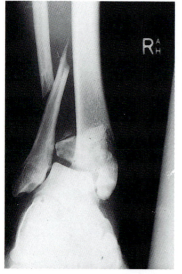

128.

a. What is the diagnosis and most likely cause?
b. What are the treatment options in a 20-year-old?
c. List the complications of this injury.

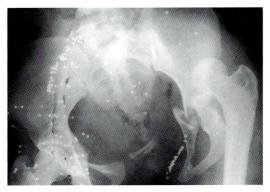

129.

a. Describe the injury in a 23-year-old African woman and give a likely cause.
b. List the important complications.
c. What are the multiple small opacities over the pelvis?

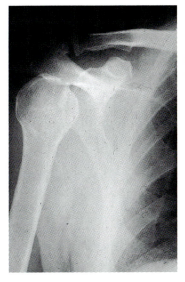

130.

a. Describe the diagnosis in the X-ray.
b. What are the clinical features?
c. How can the diagnosis be confirmed?

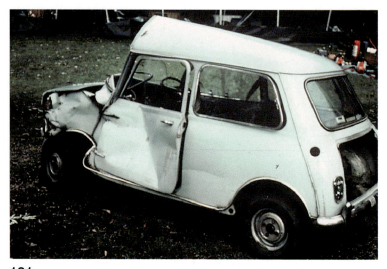

131. If seat belts and head restraints are not used in a car, describe the injuries more likely to be sustained by:

a. Driver.
b. Front seat passenger.

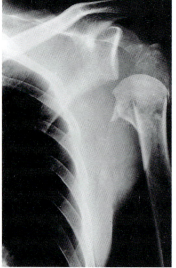

132.

a. What is the diagnosis of this condition in a young man?
b. What complications should be looked for?
c. How should this be treated?

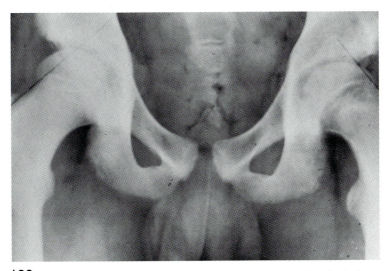

133. **A boy aged 11 presents with pain in his hip after jumping on a trampoline.**

a. What is the diagnosis?
b. What are the likely clinical signs?
c. What treatment can be proposed?

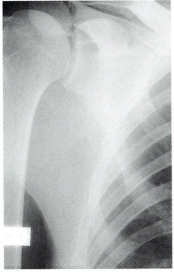

134.

a. Name the injury seen here.
b. Is the injury recent or old?
c. How may this fracture be simply treated?

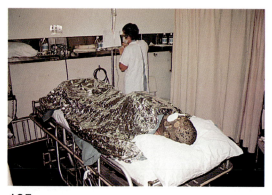

135.

a. Why was this patient admitted to hospital?
b. Outline a simple fluid therapy regime.
c. What are the common complications of this injury?

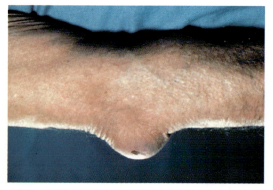

136.

a. Name the eponym by which this condition is known and give two other sites where this type of lesion can occur.
b. What is the likely cause?
c. Outline a simple plan of management.

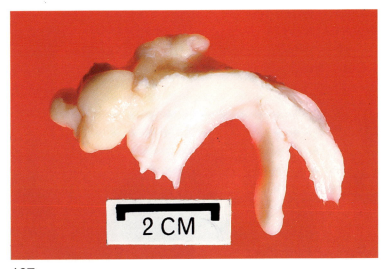

137. A tear of the medial meniscus including the 'posterior horn' — the so-called parrot-beak tear excised in the past by open operation and now by arthroscopic meniscectomy.

a. Describe the mechanism of injury.
b. What is useful in the clinical history?
c. Name other structures that may have been damaged in the knee.

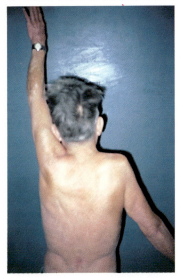

138. An elderly man presents with pain on abducting his right arm and a history of a fall onto his shoulder.

a. What is the differential diagnosis of this man's condition?
b. He can abduct his arm to 30°— how does he achieve this movement?
c. How would you substantiate your diagnosis?

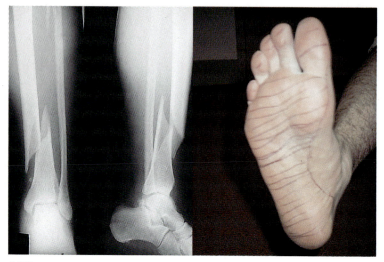

139.

a. What is the diagnosis from the X-ray and photograph?
b. What is the nerve most likely to be injured in this fracture?
c. What deficit will occur with this complication?

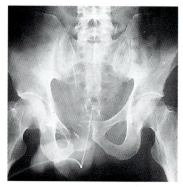

140. A patient sustained these injuries after a fall from a height.

a. Describe this X-ray.
b. Describe the various treatment options for this type of injury depending upon the severity.
c. Give the major complication and list other important problems of the injury.

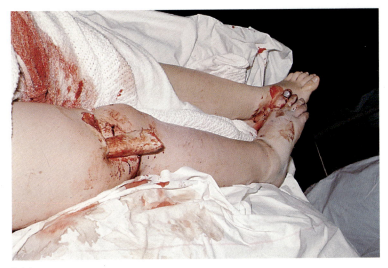

141.

a. What is your first priority in the management of this patient?
b. What are the important local complications of this injury?

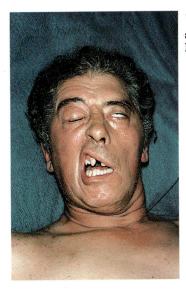

142. This elderly man suffered a fractured base of the skull. Describe the residual deformity.

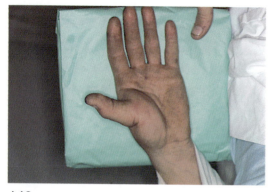

143.

a. What is the diagnosis?
b. Name possible complications of this injury.
c. Does this commonly occur?

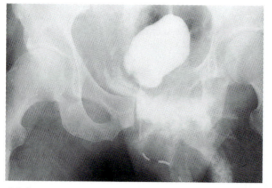

144.

a. What is the diagnosis?
b. What clinical signs may be evident?
c. Summarise the treatment of this patient.

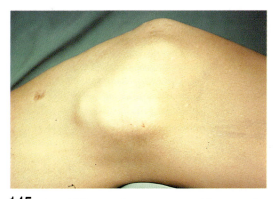

145. A middle-aged man gave a history of a severe injury to the medial side of the right knee 6 months ago. He now has a slightly painful, hard and irregular swelling on the medial side of the joint.

a. What is the most likely cause of the swelling?
b. Where does it occur?

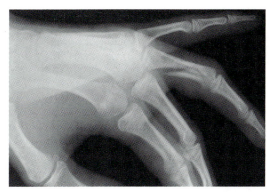

146.

a. How would you manage this patient?
b. What is the main complication?
c. If the fracture involves the articular surface, how could your treatment differ?

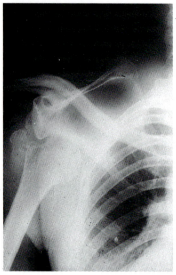

147.

a. What is the diagnosis?
b. Discuss the position of the limb and mechanism of injury.
c. What are the possible complications of the injury and the reduction?

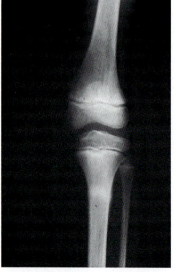

148. A new army recruit gave a history of pain over his upper tibia following an unaccustomed march.

a. Describe the X-ray.
b. What is the diagnosis?

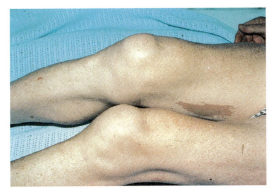

149.

a. Describe the diagnosis in an elderly patient who slipped on a carpet.
b. Is surgical repair necessary?
c. How may this patient have presented if 40 years younger?

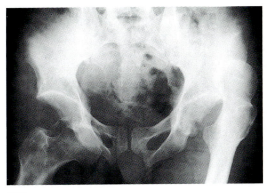

150.

a. What is the diagnosis?
b. Describe some complications.

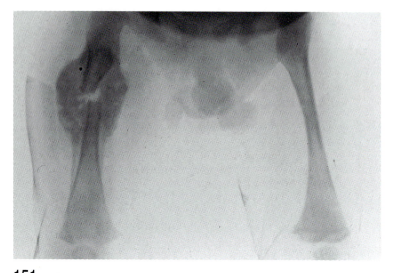

151. This baby's mother has severe diabetes.

a. How was this trauma caused?
b. Describe the features seen on this X-ray.
c. Give a brief description of how fractures heal.

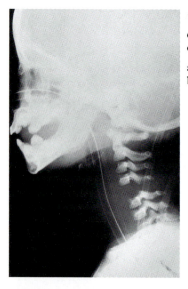

152. This is the X-ray of the cervical spine of a 2-year-old child hit by a truck.

a. What is the diagnosis?
b. Is the prognosis good or poor, and why?

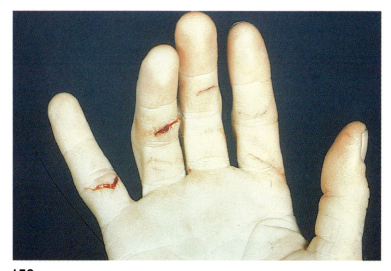

153. Late on a Saturday night, in a busy casualty department, you attend to this young male with injuries to his hands. Why is this a serious injury?

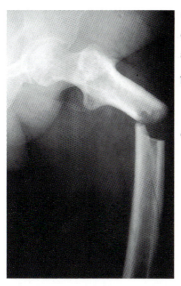

154. This is an X-ray of a closed fracture of the femur.

a. What does the term 'closed' mean?
b. Would blood loss be limited, and if so would an intravenous drip and blood cross match be unnecessary?
c. More X-rays should be taken of the injury. What are they?

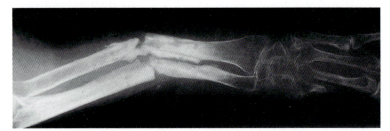

155.

a. Describe this X-ray.
b. What further complications may occur?
c. How would you treat this injury?

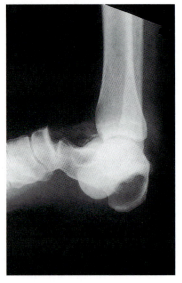

156.

a. What is the diagnosis?
b. Discuss the treatment.
c. List the complications of this injury.

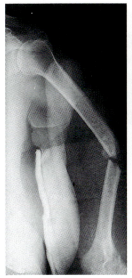

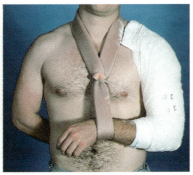

157.

a. What abnormality can be seen?
b. Name the nerve most likely to be involved.
c. Does this fracture need internal fixation?

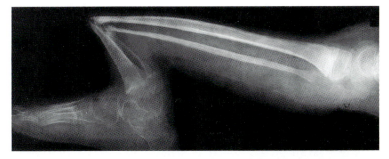

158. A 5-year-old child presents with a fracture of the tibia and fibula of several months' duration. X-rays of the pelvis show various deformities.

a. Describe the X-rays
b. What is the likely cause?

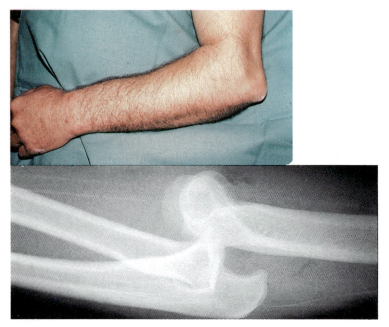

159.

a. What abnormality can be seen?
b. Discuss the mechanism of injury.
c. Outline a plan of management.

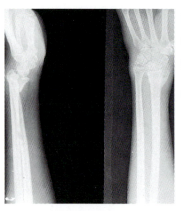

160.

a. What name is given to this particular fracture?
b. Outline how you would treat this patient.
c. List the important complications.

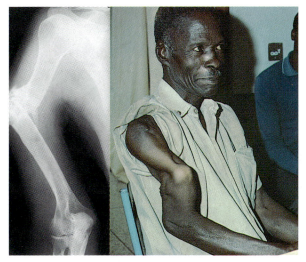

161.

a. What deformity does this X-ray show?
b. Discuss a method for correcting this problem.
c. List several causes of delayed union following a fracture.

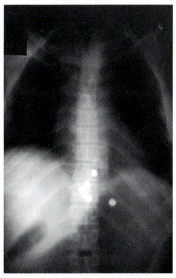

162. **A 40-year-old African man attended hospital for the first time with a history of trauma to his back.**

a. What is the cause of his injury?
b. What are the likely complications?

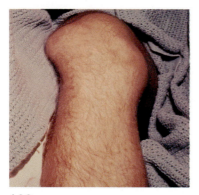

163.

a. What is the diagnosis?
b. Outline your management.
c. List the underlying conditions predisposing to this condition.

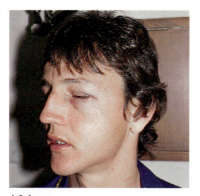

164. This man was involved in a brawl at a pub.

a. Name the structure that has been fractured here.
b. What is a common cause of this fracture?
c. What late complication may occur?

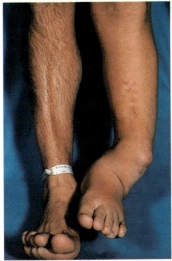

165.

a. What is the cause of this deformity?
b. Is any treatment required?
c. What problem is likely to occur at
   the knee and ankle in the future
   if this deformity is not corrected?

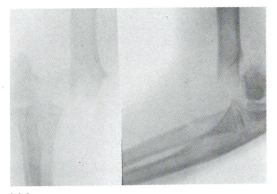

166.

a. What is the diagnosis?
b. List the main complications of this injury.
c. What age group is commonly affected?

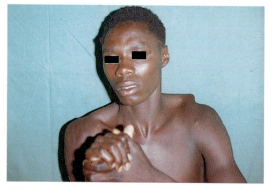

167.

a. What abnormality can be seen?
b. What is the likely cause?
c. What is the usual treatment?

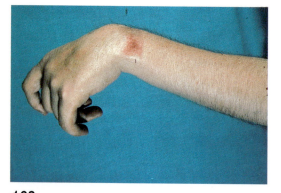

168. **A 30-year-old man who sustained a fractured shaft of the humerus 3 months earlier now has this picture.**

a. What structure has been injured?
b. Where on his upper limb may the trauma have occurred?
c. Describe the sensory loss to this hand.

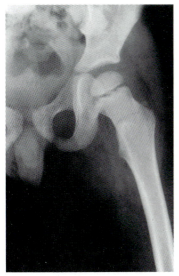

169. An 8-year-old boy presents after a fall off his bicycle.

a. What abnormality can be seen in this X-ray?
b. Give two alternative methods of treatment in this case.

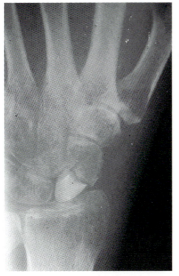

170.

a. What is the complication seen on this X-ray?
b. What other complication is likely in the future?

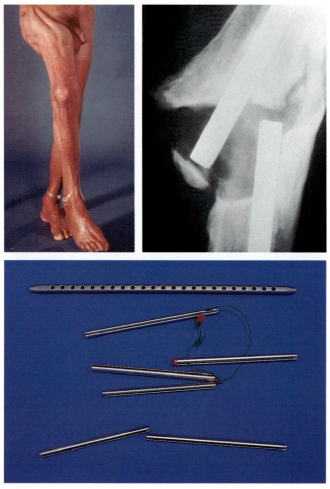

171.

a. What is the underlying diagnosis of this deformity?
b. There were three broken Kuntscher nails over a 9-year period. Why should this have happened?
c. How should this be treated?

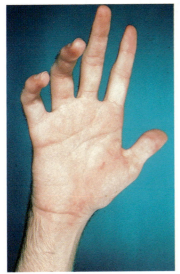

172.

a. What is the cause of this deformity?
b. What motor test can demonstrate other muscle involvement which will help confirm the diagnosis?
c. What sensory area may be affected?

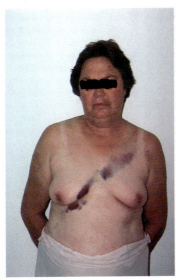

173.

a. Discuss the injury sustained by this patient and why did it occur?
b. List the many complications of this injury.

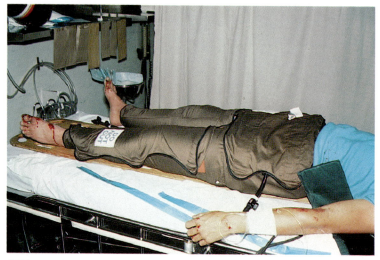

174.

a. What are these trousers called and what are they used for?
b. What precautions must be taken?

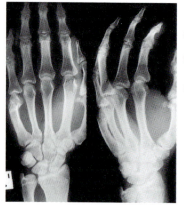

175.

a. What name is given to this common fracture?
b. How should this patient be treated?
c. With what residual deformity will the patient be left?

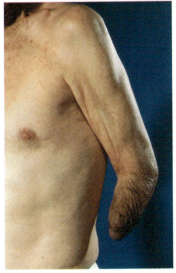

176. **This man has had a below elbow amputation of his left arm.**

a. List the common indications for this.
b. Discuss some important early and late complications.
c. Will the patient ever feel that the hand is still present and how is this minimised?

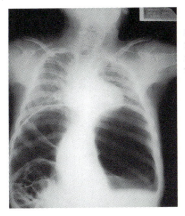

177. **An AP X-ray of the chest and abdomen in a 40-year-old male who was involved in a motor cycle accident. What is the diagnosis?**

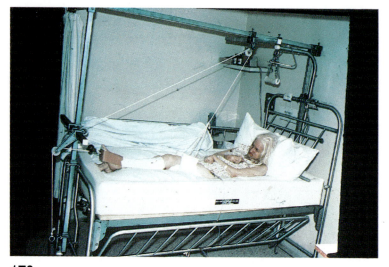

178. **An elderly female in traction for a fractured neck of femur.**

a. Which common complications may occur?
b. How are these complications best avoided?

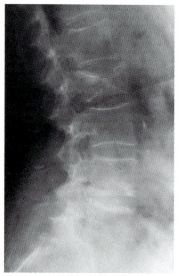

179.

a. What abnormalities can be seen?
b. How is this injury usually treated?

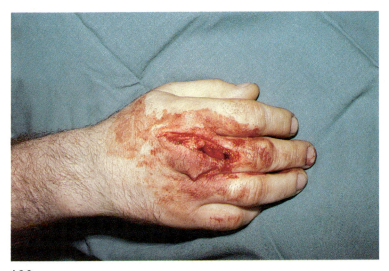

180. This middle-aged male presented at the casualty department following an accident at a factory.

a. Describe the photograph.
b. List the structures likely to be damaged.
c. What examinations would you make to evaluate the damaged structures?

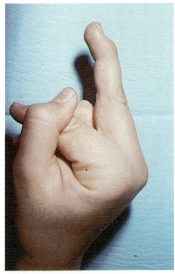

181. A young male basketball player injured his left hand while attempting to catch a ball.

a. Name this deformity.
b. How is it commonly treated?
c. Describe the method of injury.

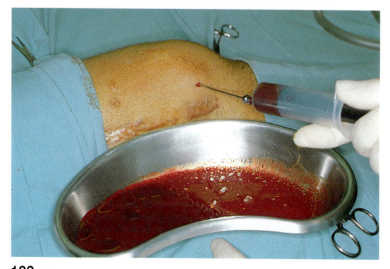

182. **A 20-year-old male injured his knee in a skiing accident.**

a. What is the diagnosis?
b. Discuss the differential diagnosis?

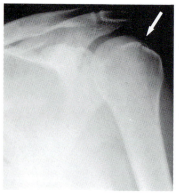

183.

a. Describe the X-ray.
b. Give a likely mechanism of injury and common complications.
c. What age group is commonly affected?
d. Discuss the treatment for this fracture.

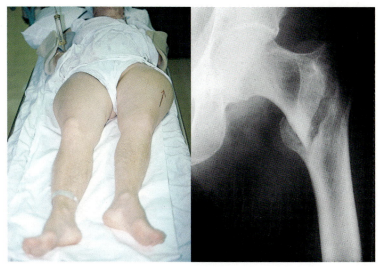

184.

a. What is the diagnosis?
b. How can this be differentiated clinically from a subcapital hip fracture?
c. Describe the position of the limb.

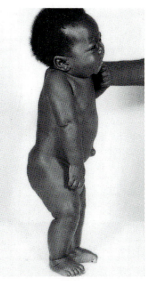

185.

a. Describe the position of this child's arm.
b. What is the cause?
c. Name the eponym by which this condition is known.
d. What is the prognosis?

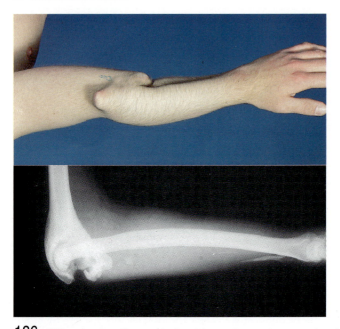

186. What is the diagnosis in this patient who sustained an injury to his arm?

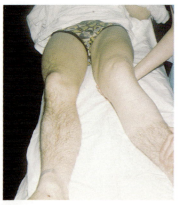

187.

a. Name the structure which has been disrupted.
b. List the triad of injuries likely to have occurred.

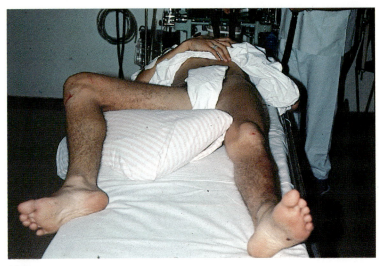

188.

a. What is the diagnosis? Comment on why an X-ray is necessary.
b. How would you treat this patient?
c. Is this injury common or rare, and what is the commonest acute complication?

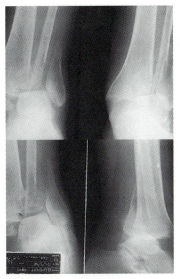

189.

a. Describe this fracture.
b. Will this fracture require internal fixation?
c. List the common complications of this injury.

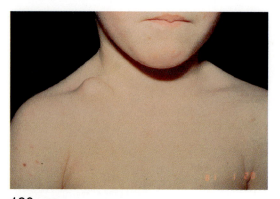

190. **This young boy has had a painful deformity over his clavicle for 2 years.**

a. What is the likely diagnosis in this case?
b. Give an explanation for your diagnosis.

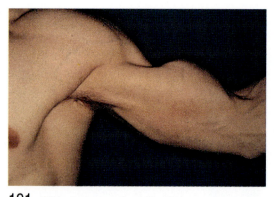

191. **This happened while lifting a bucket of water.**

a. Describe the deformity and its cause.
b. Does it require treatment?

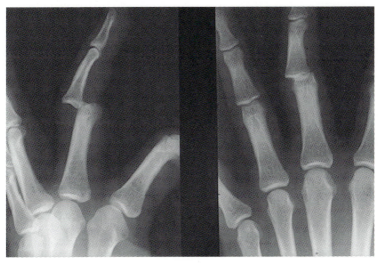

192.

a. What is the diagnosis?
b. How would you manage this patient?

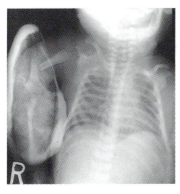

193. A baby is brought into hospital following treatment by his local doctor.

a. What is the diagnosis and how has the baby been treated?

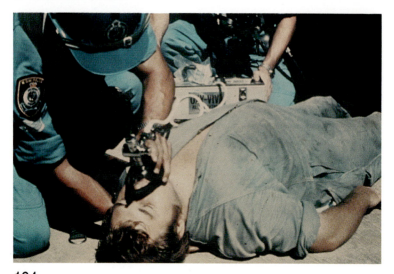

194. List the possible causes in this unconscious patient.

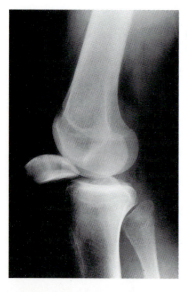

195. What is the diagnosis of this unusual condition in a 17-year-old boy?

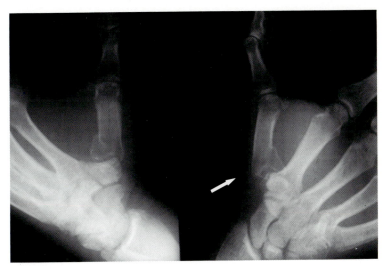

196.

a. What is the diagnosis?
b. Describe the technique of reduction.
c. What is the radio-opaque structure at the metacarpo-phalangeal joint of the thumb?

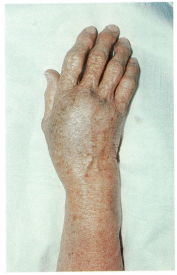

197. **A 60-year-old lady presents after fending off an attacker and injuring her right hand.**

a. What is the most likely diagnosis?
b. Is this fracture stable or unstable, and why?
c. What treatment can be offered?

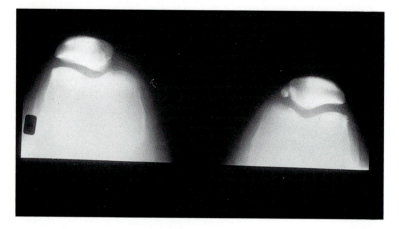

198.

a. Describe this X-ray.
b. What is the likely cause?
c. What is the differential diagnosis?

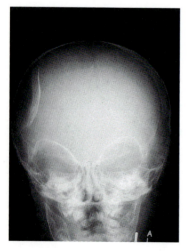

199.

a. What injury is shown?
b. Name the structure that is classically damaged with this type of fracture.
c. Outline your neurological evaluation, and likely treatment.

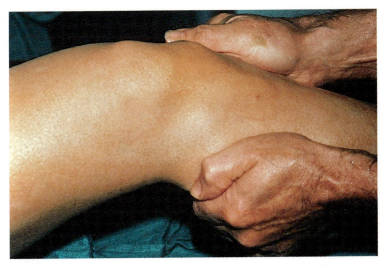

200.

a. What sign is being demonstrated here?
b. What is the underlying pathology?
c. Discuss the management for the younger and older patient.

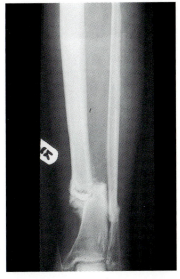

201.

a. Is this fracture new or old?
b. What are the clinical signs for union of a fracture?

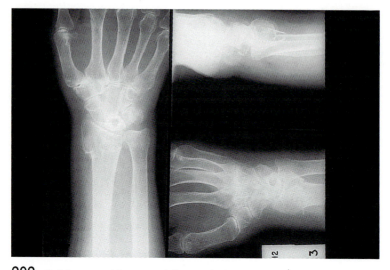

202. A 35-year-old man with a painful wrist of 2-years duration with a history of a recent fall.

a. Describe the X-ray.
b. What is the likely cause of his painful wrist?

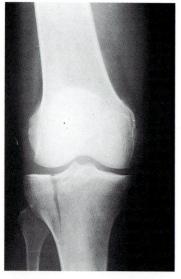

203.

a. Describe this fracture.
b. How may this have happened?
c. Outline your immediate and further treatment of this patient.

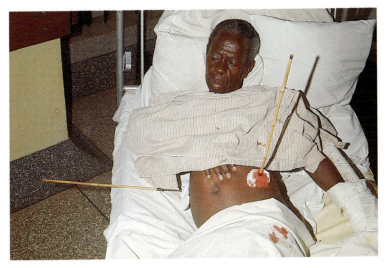

204. A middle-aged man presents with these two spear wounds in his abdomen.

a. List the possible structures that may be damaged.
b. What are your priorities in management of this patient?

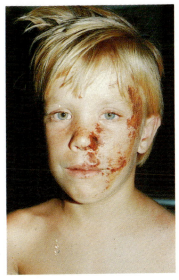

205.

a. What are the clinical signs shown in this child following trauma?
b. Name the syndrome and how it was caused.
c. How will the skin of the left forehead feel compared to the right?

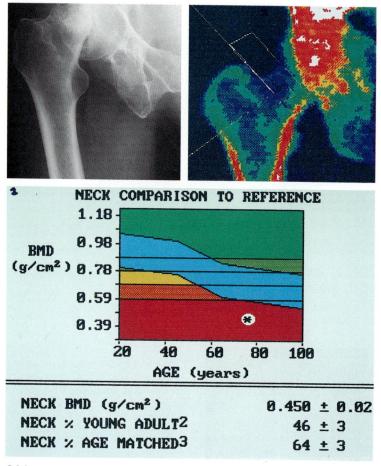

NECK BMD (g/cm²)	0.450 ± 0.02
NECK % YOUNG ADULT[2]	46 ± 3
NECK % AGE MATCHED[3]	64 ± 3

206.

a. What is the diagnosis and likely age and sex of this patient?
b. What is the main contributing factor for this condition and what treatment should be advocated?
c. What special investigation is shown?

Answers—Orthopaedics

1.
   a. Severe osteoarthritis, avascular necrosis, rheumatoid arthritis and some fractures of the neck of femur.
   b. X-ray features: osteophytes, narrowing of the joint space, subarticular sclerosis and bone cysts with avascular changes.
   c. An elderly patient with pain in the groin sometimes radiating down to the knee and a long history of repetitive injury to the joint. There is pain on exertion, relieved by rest. Flexion, adduction and external rotation deformity with restriction of movements are present, with apparent and true shortening of the affected leg.
   d. Conservative treatment includes analgesia, anti-inflammatory agents, physiotherapy and exercises. Surgical options are osteotomy or arthrodesis in the younger patient, and joint replacement in most severe cases.

2.
   a. Gouty polyarthritis—an inflammatory disorder of joints caused by the deposition of radiotranslucent monosodium urate crystals in and around joint spaces. Gout is essentially a disorder of purine metabolism, characterised by hyperuricaemia and recurrent attacks of synovitis from urate crystal deposition.
   b. Treatment consists of anti-inflammatory drugs, uricosuric agents and resting the joint. Joint effusion may require aspiration. Large deposits of urates may require operative excision.

3.
   a. Prepatellar bursal effusion.
   b. Classically called 'housemaid's knee'. People who work on their knees develop this condition, especially carpet layers working on high-friction surfaces. 'Clergyman's knee' is an infrapatellar bursitis. Gout may occasionally be responsible. A 'suprapatellar bursa' is not the bursa but merely an extension of the knee joint above the patella due to an effusion.
   c. Aspiration or surgical drainage, strapping and antibiotics for infection. A significant recurrence rate often necessitates excision of the bursal sac.

4.
   a. Dupuytren's contracture of the limbs and feet. Thickening of the palmar and digital fascia involving the skin and eventually causing contractures, mainly of the fourth fingers (sometimes all of the fingers) and toes.
   b. Surgical excision may be necessary for symptomatic

contractures. Recurrence is common and amputation of the
fifth digit may become necessary.

c. It is associated with drugs given for epilepsy, as well as in
cirrhosis of the liver, alcoholism, diabetes and pulmonary
tuberculosis. In many cases no cause is found.

5.
a. Multiple myeloma. Bone scans may sometimes be negative
in myeloma due to the extensive bone destruction. Features
include weakness, bone pain, nerve root pain, paraplegia,
anaemia and renal failure.

b. Full blood count, ESR, urinary analysis for Bence–Jones
proteose, electrophoresis and bone marrow biopsy. The
ESR was 140 mm/hour and electrophoresis revealed a peak
of globulin in the plasma. Bone marrow biopsy showed a
plasma cell dyscrasia (IgA).

c. Radiotherapy and chemotherapy plus a spinal brace are the
usual treatments. Spinal cord compression will require
urgent decompression, and fracture and potential fractures
of long bones will require operative stabilisation.

6.
a. Elongated long bone tumour with Codman's triangles and
periosteal 'onion skin' layering on one cortex and bony
spiculation (sun-burst) appearance of a fine nature on the
other side.

b. Osteogenic sarcoma with a differential diagnosis of Ewing's
sarcoma.

c. Further investigations of the leg would involve CT and
MRI scans, and radioisotope scans. A biopsy should always
be performed. A CT scan of the chest, together with a
skeletal survey and bone scan should be performed to
exclude metastases. The latest treatment for osteogenic
sarcoma is pre-operative chemotherapy for 3 months
followed by amputation or prosthetic replacement. Further
chemotherapy for 1–2 years is then usually required.

7.
a. Köhler's disease—osteochondritis of the epiphysis of the
navicular occurring in children between 2 and 9 years of
age. Characteristically, sclerosis, flattening and
fragmentation of the navicular are seen.

b. Painful limp and swelling over the navicular with
tenderness. Symptoms usually settle within a few months
with a foot support. The prognosis is excellent and within
2 to 3 years the navicular usually appears normal.

8.
a. Congenital hypothyroidism (cretinism) produces severe
dwarfism and mental retardation. The acquired form of
hypothyroidism is characterised by dwarfism and precocious
puberty.

b. Irregular epiphyseal development occurs. In this case both hips were replaced for severe degenerative osteoarthritis in bilateral dysplastic hips. Other features of hypothyroidism include a dull facies, sparse hair, dry skin, impaired mental capacity, and carpal and tarsal tunnel syndromes.

9.
a. Paget's disease (osteitis deformans) with secondary arthritis of the right hip. There is a locking intramedullary nail in the left femur to immobilise an associated fractured femoral shaft. The disease is characterised by bone resorption and formation.
b. There may be headache and deafness due to nerve compression, other nerve compressions, spinal stenosis, kyphosis, osteoarthritis, cardiac failure, hyperuricaemia and osteogenic sarcoma. Increasing bowing of the long bones is due to small cortical stress fractures. High output cardiac failure is due to multiple arteriovenous fistulae.

10.
a. The investigation is a barium swallow.
b. The patient complained of dysphagia and neck pain.
c. The patient has cervical spondylosis with large anterior osteophytes on C·4 and C·5 encroaching on the oesophagus.

11.
Inequality of foot length is usually due to a disorder at birth such as talipes equinovarus, or spinal dysraphism. It may be acquired in childhood due to conditions such as poliomyelitis or lower limb paralysis due to injury. A careful neurological examination, including examination of the spine, should be performed.

12.
a. Chronic osteomyelitis of the tibia with sinus formation. It may be post-traumatic, post-operative, follow acute osteomyelitis or be of insidious onset due to a low-grade infective organism. Typically the X-rays show areas of bone rarefaction surrounded by dense sclerosis with occasionally sequestra. Brodie's abscess, fungal infection, syphilis, yaws and chronic non-suppurative osteomyelitis may be low grade from the start of the infection.
b. Appropriate antibiotics and excision of dead bone (sequestrectomy). Long-standing infection may be impossible to cure.

13.
a. A secondary malignant bone tumour from a carcinoma of the breast. The most likely primary tumour is chondrosarcoma which this proved to be.
b. Other possible tumours in the young include Ewing's sarcoma, and in older patients malignant fibrous histiocytoma and multiple myeloma. Infection due to

pyogenic arthritis with osteomyelitis is unlikely due to the length of history and lack of sinuses.

14. Gout is the diagnosis. This responded dramatically to non-steroidal anti-inflammatory drugs.

15.
a. Calcification of the articular cartilage and the menisci. Long-standing cases such as this develop secondary osteoarthritis with spur formation.
b. Chondrocalcinosis (or pseudogout) is sometimes a familial condition, where calcium pyrophosphate dihydrate crystals are deposited in joint tissues. It may be asymptomatic or resemble gout. Gout mainly affects the small joints, and chondrocalcinosis the large joints.
c. Idiopathic, or associated with hyperparathyroidism, haemochromatosis, gout and diabetes.
d. Treat as for gout with rest and anti-inflammatory drugs.

16.
a. Psoriatic arthropathy.
b. Sacroiliitis and/or ankylosing spondylitis.
c. Yes: 60% of cases are positive for HLA-B27, but this is non-specific.
d. Non-steroidal anti-inflammatory drugs and immunosuppressive agents such as methotrexate for resistant forms.

17.
a. The girl has acute rheumatoid arthritis.
b. Observe the swelling of the wrists, metacarpo-phalangeal and proximal interphalangeal joints. The left elbow and right knee also have flexion deformities.
c. Rashes, malaise, lymphadenopathy and hepatosplenomegaly.
d. Complications: ankylosis of joints, growth defects and fractures from disuse osteoporosis.

18.
a. The X-ray shows a compressed and irregular lunate bone with increased density and mottling with secondary osteoarthritis.
b. Kienböck's disease. This is due to an avascular necrosis of the lunate bone with localised tenderness. It occurs usually between the ages of 15 and 40 years, in the dominant wrist of adult male manual labourers, and may be due to trauma. It is also more common in cerebral palsy.

19.
a. Bilateral winging of the scapula—in this case congenital fascioscapulohumeral muscular dystrophy as this is bilateral and in a child.
b. The differential diagnosis of a winged scapula includes viral infections of the 5th to 7th cervical nerve roots, brachial plexus injuries and injury to the long thoracic nerve (C5,6,7).

20.

a. Osteopetrosis (Albers–Schönberg disease)—an inherited generalised skeletal dysplasia of unknown origin. The bones are marble-like and break easily. Cranial nerve palsies and pituitary fossa compression occur, as well as back pain and sciatic nerve compression. There are two forms:
   - *tarda (autosomal dominant)*, the benign form which has a normal life expectancy
   - *congenita (recessive)*, which is rare and patients rarely survive beyond 20 years as they usually die from progressive anaemia, paralysis or infection.

b. Bone marrow transplants have been used successfully.

21.

a. Achilles tendon xanthomata, calcaneal bursitis and gouty tophus overlying the tendo Achillis as in this case. Gout is likely due to the irregularity of the lump.

b. Aspiration of the lump should reveal befringent crystals and there may be an elevated serum uric acid. On examination the patient may also have gouty tophi of the ears, elbows, knees or big toe.

22.

a. The picture shows a large, diffuse vascular mass. The differential diagnosis would include malignant tumours of bone such as a Ewing's sarcoma, as this was, an osteogenic sarcomata or a metastasis from a malignant tumour. Chronic osteomyelitis is a possibility but there is no sinus and the pus is sterile.

b. An immediate X-ray and biopsy of the lesion is essential. In this case amputation (Fig. 22A) was instituted, with postoperative chemotherapy for metastatic disease.

23.

a. Leprosy involving the hands with wasting of the interossei and thenar muscles, early clawing of the left hand, loss of thumb opposition on the right, stiff fingers and absorption of several digits. These lesions are associated with ulnar and median nerve involvement. The associated loss of sensation causes ulceration. Leprosy is caused by infection with *Mycobacterium leprae*, a chronic infectious disease which predominantly affects skin, mucous membranes and nerves.

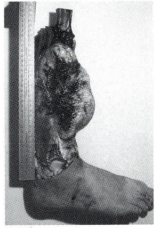

Fig 22A

b. Treatment includes chemotherapy, and tendon transfers to treat hand deformities such as clawing and loss of thumb opposition. Pressure sores under the feet may require special padded footware and sometimes operation for osteomyelitis.

24.
a. Osteogenesis imperfecta—a heterogenous disorder inherited with autosomal dominant or recessive pattern.
b. This condition is characterised by bone fragility, blue sclera, poor dentition and hearing abnormalities. The patient may sustain multiple fractures leading to progressive deformities. Scoliosis develops in adolescence and may lead to death in the older patient. There may be atlantoaxial instability from odontoid hypoplasia. This condition has been classified into various types:
- the dominant type which presents later in childhood with or without blue sclera
- the lethal variety which presents early and is associated with multiple severe fractures and progressive deformity.

25.
a. Neurofibromatosis (von Recklinghausen's disease)—a congenital condition which occurs in 1 in 3000 of the population. Half are inherited as an autosomal dominant, and the other half are new mutations.
b. Clinical manifestations are numerous: café-au-lait spots (more than 5 is virtually diagnostic) and cutaneous nodules, naevus elephantiasis, pseudoarthrosis of the tibia and hypertrophy of single limbs. Complications include progressive scoliosis, paraplegia due to neurofibroma of the spinal nerve roots pressing on the cord, malignant transformation to neurofibrosarcoma and increasing deformity.

26.
a. Chronic osteomyelitis of the lower femur.
b. Massive osteomyelitic involucrum of the lower femur with a sclerotic sequestrum.
c. Pathological fracture of the lower femur; neovascular pressure by the sequestrum; septicaemia.

27.
a. Hallux rigidus of the metatarsophalangeal joint due to osteoarthritis secondary to trauma.
b. The dorsal 'bunion' is characteristic of hallux rigidus, and the wide soft shoe shows the typical dorsal bulge.

28.
a. Lateral view of a skull showing a very large osteolytic area in the anterior half of the skull which is well delineated and lacks a sclerotic border. A similar but small area is seen in the occipital bone.

lacks a sclerotic border. A similar but small area is seen in the occipital bone.

b. This is the typical pattern of the active form of Paget's disease and is called osteoporosis circumscripta. A more advanced form of Paget's will show a larger skull with marked calvarial thickening, especially of the outer table.

29. An osteogenic sarcoma of the lower radius with multiple sclerotic secondary deposits in his bones and chest.

30.
a. A 'Baker's cyst' due to a herniation of the synovia through the posterior capsule secondary to osteoarthritis with a synovial effusion.

b. Treatment of the osteoarthritis. Excision of the cyst alone usually leads to a recurrence.

31.
a. The median nerve.

b. Carpal tunnel syndrome.

c. Conservative treatment includes rest and non-steroidal anti-inflammatory drugs. If neurological deficit is apparent, surgical release of the carpal tunnel is indicated either open or by arthroscopic decompression.

32.
a. Bilateral Perthes' disease (avascular necrosis) of the hips: 17% of all cases are bilateral. The X-ray shows flattening and fragmentation of the femoral epiphyses with increased density and a widened joint space. This typically affects young boys aged 4–10 years.

b. The symptoms may be minimal, with only a slight pain and a limp. The hip is slightly painful and irritable, with limited abduction and internal rotation, especially in flexion.

c. Russell skin traction in the acute stage, followed by an abduction splint. Osteotomy of the upper femur is sometimes necessary to contain the flattened head in the acetabulum. Late osteoarthritis is common.

33.
a. This X-ray shows a densely sclerotic vertebral body due to secondary spread from the prostatic cancer.

b. Deposits from carcinoma of the breast and bowel occasionally also give an osteosclerotic appearance. Lymphoma deposits can also mimic prostate secondaries.

34.
a. Giant cell tumour of the upper tibia (osteoclastoma). A secondary malignant deposit is the main differential diagnosis.

b. An expansive lytic lesion at the end of a long bone extending to the joint surface is characteristic of giant cell tumours. Frequently there are trabeculae and a 'soap-bubble' appearance. About one-third of such tumours are benign, one-third are usually invasive and one-third metastatic. Patients are usually aged 20–40 years and female, and present with pain (sometimes a pathological fracture), swelling or inflammation of the adjacent joint.

c. Recurrence (50%) after currettage alone, metastases and malignant transformation (10%).

d. Small lesions require curettage, cryotherapy and bone grafting. Large lesions such as this may require complete excision and bone or prosthetic replacement or, alternatively, radiotherapy and/or amputation if surgical reconstruction is impossible.

35.
a. A spondylolisthesis at the L4/5 level with a 'step' where the L4 vertebra is displaced forward on L5.
b. A congenital defect of the pars interarticularis of both pedicles of L4 allowing the vertebra to dislocate forward.
c. The most typical site is one vertebra lower with a forward slip of L5 on S1. The presence of a defect in the pars interarticularis in a vertebra above L4 is unusual.

36.
a. Widening of the epiphysis at the distal femur and proximal tibia, and a widening of epiphyses of the lower radius and ulna. There is also beaking at the margins of the epiphyseal plates.
b. Rickets.

37.
a. The patella is enlarged, slightly sclerotic and has lost its normal trabeculae.
b. Paget's disease of the patella. The long history, and the homogeneous appearance of the patella are against a diagnosis of a secondary deposit from carcinoma of the prostate. The curved femur and tibia on the opposite side are suggestive of Paget's disease.

38.
a. Massive bilateral anterior bowing of both tibiae.
b. Congenital abnormality.
c. Nothing. He would lose his livelihood as a beggar, and he and his family could die of starvation in the future.

39.
a. Ehlers–Danlos syndrome.
b. This syndrome has multiple clinical forms (nine types have been described). Enzyme defects and defects of collagen synthesis have been found in some of these types. The features include: joint hypermobility, as shown by the excessive dorsiflexion of the foot; skin laxity; a tendency to bruise leaving pigmented 'tissue paper' scars (as on this boy's legs); destructive arthropathy of the thumb; flat feet.

40.
a. A fixed thoracolumbar idiopathic scoliosis in an adolescent which is convex to the right. This deformity does not correct with forward flexion as there is structural rotation of the vertebrae with bony changes.
b. The extent of the curve must be carefully documented. Milder curves may be held with spinal braces, but surgical correction and spinal fusion is required for severe and progressive deformities.

41.
a. Achondroplasia—short-limbed dwarf with a near normal spine. The limbs are short in relationship to the trunk, e.g. the 'dachshund' of humans. Achondroplastic dwarfs are the most common type of dwarf—the so-called circus clown and strong man.
b. Autosomal dominant.
c. A large and bradycephalic skull (the head is hydrocephalic to the face), with normal intelligence. The face has frontal bossing and a saddle nose. The limbs are short (especially the proximal segments), and the trident fingers are almost equal in length. There may be kyphosis, lumbar lordosis, disc rupture and spinal stenosis causing paralysis. The lumbar lordosis and waddling gait give the appearance of hip dislocation, and the hip and other joints may be dysplastic.

42.
a. Pes planus (flat foot). Loss of the medial arch of the foot with a valgus heel and pronation of the forefoot.
b. Anatomical and physiological causes have been described. The former include external rotation of the leg, genu valgum, equinus deformity, varus forefoot deformity, congenital 'rocker-bottom' foot and spasmodic and paralytic flat foot.
c. A hypermobile and pain-free flat foot requires no treatment except for a longitudinal arch support in the elderly with symptoms. Spasmodic flat foot due to congenital subtaloid fibrous or bony bar may require a walking cast or surgical excision of any abnormal bony bridges. Subtaloid or triple arthrodesis may be necessary in some cases.

43.
a. Solitary lytic metastasis to femur with cortical erosion and endosteal scalloping, most likely from a carcinoma of the breast.
b. Surgical fixation to prevent subsequent fracture. In this case a Huckstep titanium locking intramedullary nail has been used with methyl methacrylate bone cement. This must always be followed by radiotherapy to the lesion, plus hormones and chemotherapy if indicated.

44.
a. Knuckle pads—thickenings over the dorsum of the proximal interphalangeal joints.
b. These are manifestations of Dupuytren's contracture, which is an autosomal dominant condition.

45.
a. The most likely diagnosis is a bone tumour, and at this age a secondary deposit or a chondrosarcoma of the scapula.
b. The scar is from a biopsy which confirmed the diagnosis of a chondrosarcoma.
c. Surgical excision is required for a chondrosarcoma, as these are usually resistant to both chemotherapy and radiotherapy. The prognosis is fairly good provided metastases have not already occurred.

46.
a. Macromelia (gigantism) of the entire limb, with a 46 cm long foot. In gigantism there is congenital hypertrophy of all tissue elements involved. Other forms of this congenital anomaly may involve hypertrophy of less significant proportions. These may affect a foot, toes or a single toe only, but commonly the medial three toes.
b. Neurofibromatosis and haemangiomatosis.
c. Severe disability required an above-knee amputation. The patient was fitted with an above-knee prosthesis.

47.
There is a radio-opaque structure in the region of the left hip. It does not have the appearance of any known orthopaedic implant. It is an artefact, in this case a pencil in the patient's pocket! The outline of the wood around the pencil 'lead' can be seen.

48.
a. The late sequelae of septic arthritis of the hip with destruction of the femoral head ('Tom Smith's disease').
b. Urgent incision, drainage, bed rest and high-dose intravenous antibiotics.

49.
a. Tophaceous gout with soft tissue deposition and ulceration of the overlying skin. There is cellulitis of the surrounding skin.
b. Classically, the metatarsophalangeal joint of the big toe.
c. Anti-inflammatory drugs, uricosuric agents and surgical excision of the tophus, if necessary.

50.
a. Aneurysmal bone cyst.
b. Fracture.
c. Curettage and bone grafting for small cysts. Such large cysts with impending fractures have been successfully treated with a nonvascularised graft from the ipsilateral fibula with Rush nail fixation, as in this case. A vascularised

graft would incorporate faster if the expertise were available to insert this.

51. Erythema ab igne. The patient has sat on the right side of her fireplace for many years. The erythema and discoloration are due to the effects of localised heat.

52.
a. A ruptured Baker's cyst—a synovial herniation from an arthritic knee joint which ruptures causing intense calf pain and swelling. This may mimic a deep vein thrombosis, but there is no ankle oedema in this case.
b. An arthrogram will demonstrate contrast leaking from the knee joint down to the calf. It is important to exclude vascular and neurological compression on the popliteal vessels or the medial popliteal nerve.
c. Treatment is symptomatic and may require arthroscopic synovectomy and shaving, and removal of eroded cartilage and loose bodies. Severe osteoarthritis of the knee usually later requires knee replacement surgery.

53.
a. Bilateral dislocation of both hips with a pathological fracture of the upper left femur. The heads are well formed, as are both acetabulae.
b. Pyogenic arthritis of both hips with dislocation and osteomyelitis of the left femur, with a fracture. Congenital dislocation of the hips (CDH), apart from the history of only one month's duration, would show poorly developed sloping acetabulae, and less well-formed heads. Traumatic dislocation of both hips is unlikely with the history of a febrile illness, and with no history of trauma.

54. A malignant tumour, in this case a fibrosarcoma infiltrating the skull. An important differential diagnosis is a secondary deposit from carcinoma elsewhere, but the length of history is against this.

55.
a. The vertebral bodies show a 'bamboo spine' with ligament ossification. This is seen in ankylosing spondylitis, a chronic inflammatory disorder characterised by synovitis of the synovial joints and inflammation at the fibro-osseous junctions of syndesmotic joints and tendons. It occurs mostly in males aged 20–30 years, affecting the spine and sacroiliac joints with pain and stiffness of the back and neck. Laboratory tests may show a raised ESR and non specific HLA-B27 present in 90% of cases.
b. There is a decrease in all spinal movements, often with kyphosis, decreased chest expansion and central joint involvement, especially the sacroiliac and hip joints. Extra-articular manifestations include ocular inflammation, aortic valve disease, carditis and pulmonary fibrosis.

56.

a. Hallux valgus deformity of the big toes with a bunion (bursa) over the medial side of the prominent first metatarsal heads. The second toe is displaced by the deviated big toe. This is the most common foot deformity, and tends to occur in older females (over 60 years).

b. Treatment includes modification of footwear with foot exercises, a bunion pad and an orthotic support. When this fails, surgical corrective osteotomy of the first metatarsal, or one of a number of other operations, is necessary to straighten the big toe and excise the exostosis.

57.

a. Acromegaly—hyperpituitarism starting in adulthood, with an excess output of growth hormone from the pituitary which increases the synthesis of insulin-like growth factors (somatomedins). The cause is usually a chromophobic or eosinophilic adenoma of the gland. It commonly presents with headaches and visual disturbances.

b. There is stimulation of bone growth in the growing child with gigantism. In the mature skeleton there is hypertrophy of articular cartilage. The jaw and skull enlarge, the hands and feet are enlarged and long bones are markedly thickened. Osteoarthritis is common, especially of the hips. Carpal tunnel syndrome may also occur.

58.

a. AIDS with extensive cutaneous Kaposi sarcomata in a homosexual man. There is the typical extensive muscle wasting of the neck, shoulder girdle and para-spinal regions which are seen in the full-blown case of HIV infection.

b. The following orthopaedic problems have occurred in AIDS patients: osteomyelitis, septic arthritis, polyarthritis, bony tumours, skin ulcers and flexion contractures. Such complications are depicted in the Figure on page 30, with a fixed flexion contracture of the knee from extensive Kaposi sarcomata in the soft tissues. Other associated conditions include: Reiter's syndrome, reactive and psoriatic arthritis, myopathies, polymyositis, paraplegia and the 'sicca' syndrome.

59.

a. The tibia and femur in Paget's disease. There is a surgical scar over the left femur after an operation for a pathological fracture.

b. Dull constant ache in the leg, worse at night, with associated deformity; pain and swelling of the knee due to osteoarthritis; hip and back pain.

c. Analgesics plus calcitonin or diphosphonates to control the disease. Treatment of complications includes internal fixation of fractures or an osteotomy to correct the deformity.

60.
a. Neonate with unilateral right congenital dislocation of hip. This condition is rare in Africa and particularly common in some countries such as Japan and Italy.
b. There is a familial incidence. It is much more common in girls than boys and, in one-third of patients, both hips are affected.
c. For a neonate, an abduction pillow or an abduction harness after reduction. Late operation may be necessary.

61.
a. Bone and a bursa over the 5th metatarsal base. It is a heterotopic bone or irritation callus due to irritation by 'flippers' worn when swimming.
b. Treatment was symptomatic. The flippers needed to be left off for several months, followed by different flippers which did not rub on his 5th metatarsals.

62.
a. Onychogryposis—a condition where the nail becomes thickened and grows to resemble a ram's horn if left uncut. It is usually precipitated by trauma or a fungal infection. It is frequently seen in unkempt patients.
b. Radical excision of the nail bed is required. If merely trimmed, the nail will grow back in the same form.

63.
a. Osteosarcoma of the proximal humerus. This is the most likely tumour in this age group, commonly occurring between 10 and 25 years of age. A second peak occurs in middle age due to a parosteal osteogenic sarcoma, and a third peak in the 60s to 70s (secondary to Paget's disease).
b. ESR, WBC count, and cultures exclude infection. Bone scan and CT lung scan to determine the presence of metastases, and biopsy to confirm the diagnosis.
c. Forequarter amputation as this tumour is too advanced for limb-sparing surgery. Prior adjuvant and subsequent chemotherapy if possible.

64.
a. Spina bifida—a defect in the neural arch where the two halves have failed to fuse. The cord or membranes may protrude with varying degrees of spinal cord involvement. It affects 3% of the population, particularly the first-born, and is familial. It may also be associated with folic acid deficiency during pregnancy.
b. A suprapubic catheter in place for bladder dysfunction, and small feet with atrophic skin.
c. Motor paralysis and sensory loss in lower limbs; loss of neurological control of bowels and bladder, kyphosis, hip dislocation, genu recurvatum, talipes equinovarus and claw toes. Hydrocephalus may also occur in severe cases.

65.
a. A cocked-up and defunct toe from a burns contracture of 6 years' duration in a 70-year-old male with epilepsy, whose foot was burnt when he had a fit in front of a fire.
b. If symptomatic the toe can be amputated.

66.
a. Cleft or lobster hands and feet in a young African. This is one of the two types of deformity involving the hand where a deep palmar cleft separates the two central metacarpals with one or two rays usually absent or fused. In lobster foot the single cleft may extend to the tarsus.
b. Surgery is usually not necessary if the hand is functional and the patient is able to walk. Surgery is only occasionally necessary on cosmetic grounds.

67.
a. The grossly deformed hands of advanced rheumatoid arthritis with ulnar deviation of the fingers and radial deviation of the wrists. There are hyperextension deformities of the fingers and dislocated right metacarpophalangeal joints. There is also marked synovial joint swelling and dislocation of the metacarpophalangeal joints, and rupture of the extensor tendons.
b. 'Z-shaped' deformity of the thumb. In rheumatoid arthritis, as a result of joint and extensor tendon destruction, instability and muscle imbalance, the thumb loses its ability to act as an effective opposition point.

68.
a. Chondrosarcoma secondary to malignant change in an osteochondroma in diaphysial aclasis. This is an autosomal dominant disorder where there is failure of bone remodelling and multiple osteochondroma.

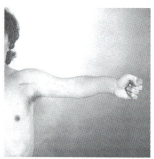

b. There were also multiple lumps on the upper humerus, lower radius and ulna, around the femora, knees, ankles and flat bones. Bowing of the radius due to insufficient development of the ulna and genu valgum were also present.

Fig 68A

c. The chondrosarcoma required wide local surgical excision and replacement with a fibular graft from his own fibula. This incorporated well and he now has a strong arm and hand with no neurological or vascular deficit (Fig. 68A). There has also been no recurrence after eleven years' follow-up.

69.
a. Congenital bilateral hypoplastic big and 5th toes.
b. There would be significant loss of power of push-off due to the absence of the big toe.
c. The patient is functioning well so no operative treatment is required.

70.
a. Paget's disease (osteitis deformans) with enlargement of the skull. The skull changes are commonly osteolytic in the vault (osteoporosis circumscripta). In the chronic osteoblastic phase there is an increase in skull size.
b. Hearing loss may be sensorineural due to cochlear dysfunction or conductive from ankylosis of the ossicles. Other symptoms include headaches and, occasionally, pressure on the optic nerve which may cause blindness. Severe disease of the skull may lead to life-threatening spinal cord compression or impingement on the brain stem. Other complications of Paget's disease include bowing and pathological fractures of long bones, kyphosis with back pain, osteoarthritis, osteogenic sarcoma and heart failure due to arteriovenous shunts in the bones.

71.
a. Bilateral genu varum of 100°, with internal torsion of both tibiae of 90°.
b. Blount's disease (adolescent tibia vara), a condition where the postero-medial part of the proximal tibial epiphysis has failed to develop as much as the lateral epiphysis.
c. Large bony wedges should be taken out of both tibiae with osteotomy of both fibulae as performed here with internal fixation with staples. The common peroneal nerves were carefully isolated and the patient was able to run and to play football after the operation (Fig. 71A).

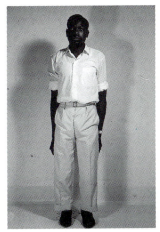

Fig 71A

72.
a. Acute pyogenic osteomyelitis and trauma (i.e. child abuse).
b. Blood cultures, ESR, WBC count and culture of the pus. Note that in the first two or three weeks of infection an

X-ray would be negative. A bone scan may also be considered. After a thorough examination, including examination of the axillary lymph glands, a skeletal survey may be carried out to reveal other fractures associated with child abuse if trauma is the cause.

73.
a. Morton's metatarsalagia (Betts' neuroma)—a painful neuroma of a digital nerve, which occurs between the metatarsal necks proximal to the division of the digital nerves to the second, third or fourth clefts. There is tenderness under the forefoot on weight bearing and on deep pressure between the heads of the 2nd and 3rd or 3rd and 4th metatarsal heads. Lateral pressure on the sides of the forefoot is also painful. The pain is worse at night when the feet are warm. It usually affects overweight women with poor muscles and is aggravated by tight shoes.
b. Anterior metatarsalgia with tenderness under the heads of the 2nd, 3rd or 4th metatarsals due to poor intrinsic muscles. This may, however, coexist with a neuroma.
c. Radical excision of the neuroma if a pad behind the anterior metatarsal heads is unsuccessful.

74.
a. Infantile torticollis due to a contracted sternomastoid muscle with secondary facial asymmetry (hemiatrophy). The eye line is higher on the left side. The torticollis may have followed a difficult labour or breech delivery.
b. Surgical release of the sternomastoid is usually required. At this late stage, correction may leave the patient with residual facial asymmetry and may adversely affect the visual axes.
c. Secondary torticollis may result from an acute disc prolapse, skin scarring, inflamed neck glands, ocular disorders, injuries of the cervical spine and congenital deformities. Spasmodic torticollis may be due to a psychological cause.

75.
a. Congenital dislocation of both hips (CDH) in the boy. Note the width of the perineum in the boy.
b. CDH is much commoner in girls.

76.
a. Chondrosarcoma of the 3rd metacarpal is the most likely diagnosis. This often arises from a pre-existing enchondroma or is associated with Ollier's disease. Enchondroma is the most common bone tumour of the hand. It usually occurs in the proximal phalanx of the digit. Exostoses are usually multiple and malignant changes to a chondrosarcoma occur in about 1% of patients. Bony infection is excluded by the absence of constitutional features and a lack of a periosteal reaction.

b. Total excision may be curative if the soft tissues have not been involved, as chondrosarcomata metastasise late.

77.
a. Bilateral genu valgum—'knock knee'.
b. Idiopathic (bilateral in young children). Other causes include bone softening (rickets, dysplasias, rheumatoid arthritis), epiphyseal injuries and fractures, osteoarthritis, ruptured ligaments, Charcot joints, paralytic conditions and fixed adducted hips due to trauma or infection.
c. A corrective varus osteotomy or epiphyseal arrest on the medial aspect of the knee with staples or by an epiphysiodesis.

78.
a. Degenerative osteoarthritis of the medial compartment of the knee, producing a varus knee.
b. Pain and stiffness on the medial side of the knee, tenderness over the medial joint line with pain on varus compression of the joint.
c. A tibial osteotomy would correct the mechanical malalignment of the joint and unload the medial compartment. In this case a total knee replacement was necessary.

79.
a. Bilateral coxa vara in a child.
b. Coxa vara may be congenital or acquired. In this case it is due to a congenital cause. Other causes of congenital varus include multiple epiphyseal dysplasia, familial osteopetrosis, achondroplasia and cretinism. Acquired causes include: childhood injury, rickets, and Perthes' disease.
c. Abnormal stresses on the hip joint and possible avascular necrosis will cause secondary osteoarthritis.

80.
a. Congenital bilateral complex syndactyly of the hands ('rose bud hands'), a congenital below-knee amputation of the left leg, flexion deformity of the right knee with a wasted retroverted leg.
b. Surgical correction plus artificial limbs. Rehabilitation allowed the child to walk, write and be educated (Fig. 80A).

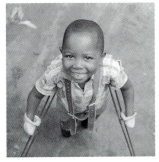
Fig 80A

81.
a. Pes cavus—a high-arched foot with a varus heel. The deformity is a result of imbalance created by the loss

of intrinsic muscles of the foot. Later, clawing of the toes may develop.

b. i. Congenital: spina bifida, Charcot–Marie–Tooth syndrome, treated club foot or Friedreich's ataxia

ii. Acquired: poliomyelitis and other paralytic causes, Volkmann's ischaemic contracture secondary to trauma.

iii. Idiopathic: familial asymptomatic and due to unknown causes.

82.
a. Paget's disease of the humerus. This condition may involve a single bone or be widespread.

b. The humerus of this man shows irregular new bone formation on the medial cortex with a lateral area of bone destruction. Alteration in the X-ray appearance and increased pain should always suggest malignant transformation to Paget's osteosarcoma, which has occurred in this case.

c. Zero 5-year survival rate.

83.
a. A ganglion of the dorsum of the wrist. Ganglia are thought to arise from small bursae within the substance of the joint capsule.

b. The wall of the cyst is composed of fibrous tissue with clear and viscous fluid. The cyst may be uniloculated or multilocular.

c. The swelling may resolve spontaneously. Symptomatic excision is best under tourniquet (Fig. 83A). Recurrence is common following the classical treatment of hitting the lump with the 'family bible'.

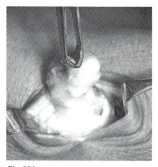

Fig 83A

84.
a. Congenital genu recurvatum, possibly related to abnormal intrauterine pressure and excessive maternal oestrogens. Occasionally also seen in arthrogryphosis or in congenitally shortened quadriceps.

b. The knees flexed to about 60° in plaster of Paris for 3 weeks for postural deformity. True congenital shortening of the quadriceps will need operative lengthening.

85.
a. Charcot's joint showing severe joint disruption with no osteopenia.

b. Absence of pain sensitivity in the hand and weakness, with spasticity in the lower limbs.

c. Syringomyelia. Other causes of Charcot's joint include syphilis (although usually lower limbs), diabetes and leprosy (peripheral joints).

86.

a. A shortened and thickened thigh, posterior bowing and shortening of the leg with enlarged first big toe.

b. Congenital abnormality of the femur with associated tibial and fibular deficiency. There are multiple cartilaginous exostoses associated with this osteochondrodystrophy, with malignant change in the proximal phalanx of the big toe to a chondrosarcoma.

c. Above-knee amputation for an essentially useless limb should be performed after biopsy of the tumour and investigation for secondary deposits, including a CT scan of the lungs.

87.

a. Secondary deposit from a carcinoma elsewhere. The differential diagnosis in this case was osteogenic sarcoma secondary to Paget's disease which is rare, but was the diagnosis in this man.

b. Above knee amputation, or radiotherapy. The prognosis is poor with a zero 5-year survival. Chemotherapy is not usually indicated in elderly patients. Note the very 'hot' region on this man's bone scan.

88.

a. Congenital absence of lateral two toes and deficiency of the lower right tibia. Note also the abnormal left toes.

b. More commonly an absent or deficient fibula is associated with absent lateral toes. The combination seen here of lateral two toes and lower tibia is unusual.

c. Surgery is required to correct the deformity and resulting instability, as well as the shortened limb. Whenever possible the foot should be reconstructed.

89.

a. Primary generalised osteoarthritis. This common form of osteoarthritis primarily affects the distal interphalangeal joints of the hands and the first metacarpo-phalangeal joint of the thumb.

b. Pain in the hands is the first symptom followed by the formation of bony swellings around the joints and later joint deformities. Typical radiological features associated are: a decrease in the joint space, subchondral bony sclerosis, osteophytes and bone cysts.

c. Heberden's nodes—bony osteophytes over the joint.

90.

a. Paget's disease of the entire radius with overgrowth and bowing.

    b. The serum alkaline phosphate is raised and hydroxyproline levels in the urine are elevated. Technetium phosphate bone scans will show considerable uptake. Other bones may be involved.

91.

a. Tuberculosis. There is destruction of the disc spaces with secondary destruction of the vertebral bodies. Metastatic tumour deposits only affect the vertebral bodies, with preservation of the disc spaces.

b. A severe gibbus deformity (kyphos) of the mid-thoracic spine, with a large abscess on the left side.

c. Pressure on the cord causing paraplegia with sensory, motor and bladder paralysis. Tuberculosis of the chest plus secondary bronchopneumonia due to diminished respiratory expansion, systemic upset and tuberculosis elsewhere.

92.

a. A pathological fracture through a typical non-ossifying fibroma of the tibia in a teenager.

b. Treat as an ordinary fracture with an above-knee plastic wrap or plaster of Paris. If it continues to enlarge, excision and grafting may be necessary.

93.

a. Flexion contractures of the wrists and hands with cylindrically shaped limbs and absent skin creases. The forearms are pronated with adduction and internal rotation of the shoulders.

b. Arthrogryposis multiplex congenita. This is a disorder characterised by stiffness of many joints, contractures, cylindrical shapeless limbs and absent skin creases. It is thought to be secondary to an intrauterine viral infection.

94.

a. Multiple flexion contractures involving the elbows, wrists, hands, hips and knees. Adduction internal rotation contracture of the shoulder with lumbar hyperlordosis. The right hand demonstrates clenched fingers with thumb in the palm posture, and extension and swan neck deformities in the left hand.

b. Her history and posture suggest a global spastic condition from birth. She has spastic tetraplegic cerebral palsy. Cerebral palsy may result from perinatal anoxia, trauma, kernicterus or infection.

c. Muscle imbalance in spastic cerebral palsy gives rise to adduction and internal rotation of the shoulder, flexion of the elbow, pronation of the forearm, flexion of the wrist, adduction of the thumb, flexion and adduction of the hips, flexion of the knees and equinus of the feet, and scoliosis. Subluxation or dislocation of the hips may occur.

95.
a. Pyogenic arthritis of the sterno-clavicular joint.
b. If high-dose intravenous antibiotics are not rapidly successful after initial blood culture and possible aspiration of the joint, incise the associated boil. Gram stain the pus, and start high-dose intravenous antibiotics. If there is no response in 48 hours, incise and drain the joint. The most likely organism is *Staphylococcus aureus* which is often resistant to penicillin. The sterno-clavicular and sacroiliac joints are often affected in drug addicts, and other joints may be infected without an obvious cause.

96.
a. Cryptococcosis (torulosis)—fungal infection of the ulna with multiple osteolytic lesions and bony destruction, and minimal periosteal reaction. The primary focus is in the lung with characteristic spread to the meninges and occasionally to the kidneys.
b. Chest, central nervous system, spine, pelvis and the major long bones.
c. HIV-positive, diabetic, TB patients, patients with sarcoidosis and those on steroid medications, i.e. patients who are immuno-compromised.

97.
a. Charcot's joint.
b. Tabes (syphilis), syringomyelia, meningocoele, diabetes, steroid injections, leprosy and lower motor or peripheral nerve paralysis.

98.
a. Marked shortening of the femur with flexion of the hip and knee and external rotation. This is the typical posture of a patient with a congenital abnormality of the femur known as a proximal femoral focal deficiency. Complete absence of the femur is rare.
b. Drugs (thalidomide), genetic inheritance, X-rays in the first 8 weeks of foetal life, rubella and unknown.
c. Gross leg length inequality, malrotation, instability of the hip joint and inadequate proximal musculature. Note also the small foot and tibia, and the deformed fingers.

99.
a. The most outstanding feature is marked kyphosis of the upper thoracic spine resulting in a grooved sternum caused by the mandible. Other deformities include flexion and adduction contractures of the hips due to spastic paraplegia.
b. Congenital. The alternative diagnosis is ankylosing spondylitis.
c. The severe kyphosis required surgical osteotomy plus spinal fusion. The flexion–abduction deformity of the hip and knee due to contracture of the ilio-tibial band was corrected by fasciotomy.

100. The differential diagnosis includes benign lesions such as fibroma, haemangioma and cartilage capped exostosis. Neurofibromatosis should be considered and café au lait spots examined for. A rhabdomyosarcoma would increase in size much more rapidly, as would secondary malignant deposits, Ewing's sarcoma, chondrosarcoma due to change in an osteochondroma and osteogenic sarcoma.

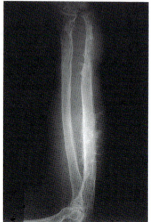

Fig 100A

In this case the slow increase in size indicates a low-grade malignant tumour and this was a multicentric fibrosarcoma causing an underlying periosteal reaction, as shown in the X-ray (Fig. 100A).

101.
a. Chronic osteomyelitis of the calcaneus. Pseudomonas infection may be responsible and cause few systemic symptoms.
b. A puncture wound of the foot is common in children. Haematogenous spread from a distant site is also a possibility and is usually caused by *Staphylococcus aureus*.
c. Radical debridement and drainage for extensive chronic osteomyelitis. Parenteral antibiotics for 3–6 weeks followed by oral antibiotics for at least 3 months.

102.
a. The head of the metatarsal has become prominent and painful due to poor intrinsic muscles of the foot.
b. Overweight elderly women with poor muscles and footwear are particularly likely to develop this condition. It is usually treated with an anterior metatarsal support behind the metatarsal heads and intrinsic muscle re-education. If operation is required, an osteotomy of the neck of the metatarsal rather than excision of the head of the bone is the best treatment.

103.
a. Congenital synostosis of the distal radius and ulna.
b. The ulna is shortened more than the radius, with ulnar

deviation of the wrist and limited rotation of the forearm with a pronation deformity.

c. Surgery is only indicated for significant disability.

104.
a. Severe paralytic scoliosis. Note he has to support his weak spine with his arms in order to sit.

b. Poliomyelitis. This disease is the most common cause of spinal deformities in the tropics and subtropics where poliomyelitis is still common.

Answers—Trauma

105.
a. There is separation of the symphysis pubis (diastasis) and the entire pelvis has been opened up like a book, giving the name a 'book fracture'. In addition, there is a fracture of the left pubic ramus and right ilium.
b. The patient should be nursed on her side on a firm mattress to 'shut the book' and reduce the fracture by traction on the right leg. Manipulation may be necessary, and in this case initial external fixateurs followed by internal fixation with plates was necessary.
c. Severe bleeding and shock may occur. This may require urgent blood transfusion and stabilisation of the pelvis initially with external fixateurs. Sciatic nerve injury caused by the upward displacement of the pelvis is also likely. A late painful complication is chronic low back pain due to disruption of the sacro-iliac joint.

106.
a. A meniscal cyst—usually associated with a tear of the lateral meniscus.
b. On palpation, the cyst is slightly tender, tense and may feel bony hard. It may disappear on flexing the knee.

107.
a. The median nerve. There is extensive wasting of the thenar eminence.
b. The sensory deficit would include the thumb, second, third and half of the fourth fingers anteriorly and their tips posteriorly. Sensation to most of the palmar aspect proximal to these fingers is lost.
c. Carpal dislocations, particularly the lunate, forearm fractures and dislocations of the elbow are all causes of median nerve damage. Carpal tunnel syndrome and penetrating trauma, such as cuts in front of the wrist, may be responsible but were not the cause in this patient.

108.
a. Posterior dislocation of the hip—flexed, adducted and internally rotated.
b. Reduction under general anaesthesia. With adequate relaxation the hip is flexed to 90°, traction is applied in the line of the femur and the leg is externally rotated and abducted.
c. • Sciatic nerve palsy.
   • Fractured posterior rim of the acetabulum.
   • Myositis ossificans.

- Avascular necrosis of head of the femur and secondary osteoarthritis.

Avascular necrosis results from disruption of the blood supply to the head of the femur, particularly the capsular vessels and to a much lesser extent in the ligamentum teres. It is much more likely to occur if the dislocation is not reduced within six hours. A total hip replacement may be necessary as a result in adults.

109.
a. Ruptured right tendo Achillis. The Simmonds' test is being performed: both calves are squeezed but only the left foot plantar flexes as the right tendo Achillis is ruptured.
b. Plantar flexion of the foot, i.e. jumping and climbing ladders would be difficult.
c. Surgical repair. Occasionally, conservative treatment alone is sufficient, with a plaster in plantar flexion for 6 weeks.

110.
a. Fracture of the proximal pole of the scaphoid. The history often includes a fall on the outstretched hand. Pain is demonstrated in the anatomical snuffbox and also by proximal pressure on the 2nd and 3rd metacarpal heads.
b. Always treat on suspicion, even if no fracture is seen on X-ray. Repeat X-ray at 3 weeks. Immobilise for 8 weeks using a scaphoid plaster or skelecast if available. Compression fixation of the scaphoid with a Herbert screw for displaced or complicated fractures.
c. Avascular necrosis of the proximal pole, non-union, associated lunate dislocation and late osteoarthritis of the wrist.

111.
a. Monteggia fracture dislocation—fracture of the proximal ulna with dislocation of head of radius.
b. In children, there may be an initially displaced greenstick fracture of the ulna because of the elasticity of the bone. This bends at the time of injury and then returns to its original shape. The radial head, however, remains dislocated. Accurate reduction is essential and, in children, is usually possible without operation. In adults, internal fixation of the ulna is usually necessary.
c. • Elbow stiffness.
   • Compartment syndrome.
   • Median nerve and brachial artery injury.
   • Myositis ossificans.

112.
a. The classification is based on the anatomical region of the fracture a) subcapital—as in this case; b) cervical and c) basal. Subcapital fractures are further classified by Garden into four stages:

    I   incomplete or impacted
    II complete without displacement of the femoral head
    III complete with partial displacement
    IV complete with full displacement of the head of the
        femur.

b. Avascular necrosis and secondary osteoarthritis may occur in as many as 50% of patients with subcapital fractures.

c. Yes—to mobilise the patient early and minimise complications.

113.

a. Colles' fracture of the lower radius and ulnar styloid of the elderly, with radial distal displacement, dorsal tilt and dorsal displacement of the distal fragment producing the classical 'dinner fork' deformity.

b. Reduction by traction, pronation, palmar flexion and slight ulnar deviation. Plaster backslab for 7 days and then a below elbow cast for 5 weeks. Full arm sling for one week and instructions on daily shoulder and finger exercises.

c. Malunion, osteoarthritis, stiffness of the fingers, wrist and shoulder. Reflex sympathetic dystrophy and rupture of the extensor pollicis longus tendon may also occur.

114.

a. Fracture of the 5th metatarsal base. Associated injury to the lateral ligament with possible fracture of the ankle.

b. The fracture is classically due to an inversion strain on the ankle with the pull of the peroneus brevis tendon on its insertion causing avulsion of the base of the 5th metatarsal.

c. A crepe bandage and crutches for 3 days followed by full weight bearing. If the fragment is markedly displaced, a walking plaster for 3 weeks may be necessary. The fracture usually unites without complication.

115.

a. An ununited fracture of the radius and ulna of four months' duration in a police dog named 'Inspector Morrison'.

b. Treatment consisted of a Huckstep titanium locking nail which resulted in early bony union.

116.

a. Supracondylar fracture of femur. The gastrocnemius muscle pulls the distal fragment posteriorly. Complications include:
    • damage to popliteal and femoral blood vessels
    • damage to the common peroneal and medial popliteal nerve
    • infection (if compound)
    • fat embolus
    • malunion or non-union with angulation and shortening
    • knee stiffness due to soft tissue adhesions of the quadriceps.

b. The fracture can be immobilised in 90° of flexion with a Thomas splint and traction with a Steinmann pin in the tibia. However, in most patients, and especially in the elderly, internal fixation with a large femoral condylar screw and plate should be carried out. This will usually allow the patient immediate post-operative weight bearing and reduce the risk of complications.

c. Children may have growth plate problems following a supracondylar fracture.

117.

a. Compound open fracture–dislocation of the tibia and fibula following a motor vehicle accident.

b. i ABCD (Airway, Breathing, Circulation, Disability).
ii Intravenous fluids, antibiotics and tetanus prophylaxis.
iii Pain relief
iv Elevate leg
The patient refused amputation. Limb salvage surgery involving orthopaedic, vascular and plastic reconstruction was successful (Fig. 117A).

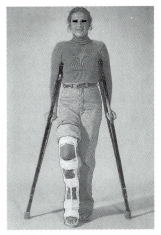

c. • Volkmann's ischaemic contracture of the calf muscles and vascular and neurological deficit.
• Non-union of fractures.
• Infection with osteomyelitis.
• Stiffness/oedema/pain.
• Late osteoarthritis.

Fig 117A

118.

a. The knee joint is dislocated.
b. The most important structures include the popliteal vessels and nerves. Associated fractures sometimes occur, and cruciate and collateral ligaments will have been damaged.
c. X-rays must be carried out to exclude fractures. Aspiration of the joint may be necessary. The orthopaedic surgeon on call must be notified early, as this is a surgical emergency and may require urgent neuro-vascular repair. A Doppler investigation and an angiogram should always be carried out to demonstrate damage to the popliteal vessels.

119.
a. This girl has cubitus valgus of her right arm, with an increased carrying angle. The deformity is seen commonly with a non-union of a fractured lateral condyle or after a supracondylar fracture, either incompletely reduced or with epiphyseal damage to the lower humerus.
b. Ulnar nerve palsy is a late complication years after the fracture. This is treated with a transposition of the nerve anteriorly and sometimes a supracondylar osteotomy to correct the deformity.
c. Cubitus varus, or the 'gun stock' deformity, shown here after malunion of a supracondylar fracture.

120.
a. Avascular necrosis of the body of the talus secondary to a fracture of the neck. The main blood supply of the talus, as with the scaphoid and head of the femur, flows from distal to proximal. A fracture of the neck of talus may therefore cut off the blood supply to the body.
b. Collapse of the talus with osteoarthritis of the ankle and subtalar joints.
c. Early internal fixation of this fracture with a compression screw, with non-weight bearing for at least 3 months. Established avascular necrosis of the body of the talus will probably require a pantalar bony arthrodesis (arthrodesis of the calcaneus to the tibia best performed with a Huckstep titanium locking compression nail).

121.
a. • Dislocated elbow.
  • Galeazzi fracture dislocation. This is a fracture of the lower radius with dislocation of the lower radio-ulnar joint.
  • Chisel fracture of the distal radius into the joint.
b. The ulnar and median nerves.

122.
a. Smith's fracture—a reversed Colles' fracture.
b. A Smith's fracture can prove difficult to reduce. It should be held in full supination and dorsiflexion in an above elbow plaster for 6 weeks or internally fixed with a T plate on the palmar aspect.
c. • Malunion.
  • Sudeck's atrophy.
  • Osteoarthritis of the wrist.

123.
a. Wasting of the muscles of the shoulder girdle with subluxation of the gleno-humeral joint, and wasting of the triceps and biceps, forearm and the small muscles of the hand. The most likely diagnosis is flail arm due to brachial plexus injury. The differential diagnosis would include an upper motor nerve lesion involving the anterior horn motor

cells such as in poliomyelitis, which has wasting but normal
sensation. In an upper motor neurone lesion such as a
stroke there is paralysis but little or no wasting or sensory
loss.
b. Most brachial plexus injuries are motorcycle accidents.
Neonatal cases are usually a traction injury during difficult
labour.
c. Fixed contractures will develop and can be avoided by
moving the limb regularly through its full range of
movements.

124.
a. This is a partially displaced oblique fracture of the midshaft
of the femur, with a lytic area around the fracture site. This
is a pathological fracture due to secondary deposits from
carcinoma of the breast.
b. Causes of a pathological fracture include:
  • metastatic tumours
  • generalised bone disease: osteoporosis, Paget's disease
  • osteomyelitis.
c. Treatment is with a Huckstep titanium locking
intramedullary nail followed by radiotherapy and hormone
therapy. Postoperative hypercalcaemia is a potentially lethal
complication in secondary deposits which must be corrected
preoperatively and watched for postoperatively.

125.
a. Myositis ossificans (traumatic ossification) due to an
unreduced dislocation of the elbow.
b. After hip dislocations, supracondylar fractures of the
humerus and prosthetic hip replacement.
c. The excessive calcification and ossification was probably
due to repeated passive stretching of the elbow in an effort
to achieve mobility, with further damage to periosteum and
muscles. Myositis ossificans is also more common in
patients with nerve and head injuries, and in those with a
predisposition to osteoarthritis.

126.
a. The 1st and 2nd toes have sustained a blade-cutting injury
with an open fracture into the 1st distal phalanx. This was
the result of the patient using a rotary blade lawn mower
while barefoot.
b. Local pressure with application of a bandage and elevation
of the limb.
c. Shock, blood loss and infection with osteomyelitis.

127.
a. Volkmann's ischaemic contracture. There is shortening of
the long flexors, flexion of the fingers, loss of bulk of the
small muscles of the hand (especially the thenar and
hypothenar eminences), fibrosis and contracture of the

forearm and an amputated fourth finger. Also note the malunion of the forearm fracture.

b. Neurological damage to the ulnar and median nerves, vascular damage and infarcted muscle, replaced by inelastic fibrous tissue.

c. Pain, paraesthesia, paralysis, pallor and a loss of pulses.

128.

a. A severely comminuted open fracture of the lower tibia and fibula due to a motor cycle injury.

b. Internal fixation to restore the stability of the joint, as shown here. Alternatively, external fixateurs (Fig. 128A), or a below knee amputation for associated severe vascular and neurological compromise. Also general treatment including tetanus toxoid prophylaxis, intravenous antibiotics and blood transfusion.

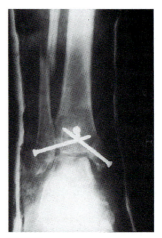

c. • Neurovascular damage.
   • Skin damage and osteomyelitis.
   • Assorted fractures and soft tissue damage.
   • Long-term deformity, stiffness and osteoarthritis.
   • Gas gangrene.

Fig 128A

129.

a. Ring fracture of the pelvis with a fracture of the left superior and inferior ischio-pubic rami, disruption of the sacro-iliac joints and dislocation of the left hip. Anterior–posterior or lateral deforming force, such as occurs in a motor vehicle accident.

b. Intra/extra-peritoneal rupture of bladder or membranous urethra, sciatic nerve injury, massive retroperitoneal haemorrhage, damage to the rectum and bowel, and osteoarthritis of the left hip. Other associated injuries include the spine, head, chest, abdomen and limbs.

c. Beads sewn into a dress of the woman which have not been removed prior to X-ray.

130.

a. There is an abnormal globular appearance of the humeral head in this AP X-ray—the typical 'light bulb' sign. The patient has a posterior dislocation of the shoulder. This is uncommon but occurs sometimes in patients with epilepsy and is often missed.

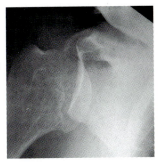

b. The arm is held internally rotated and external rotation is impossible. There may be flattening of the front of the shoulder, often obscured by swelling.

c. A lateral X-ray and a better AP X-ray (Fig. 130A) as shown, will confirm the diagnosis.

Fig 130A

131.
a. Driver—fractured sternum from the steering wheel.
b. Driver and passengers:
  • head, chest and abdominal injuries
  • fractured patella and femur
  • posterior dislocation of the hip
  • crush fracture of the thoracic and cervical spine with neurological damage
  • multiple limb fractures with neurological, vascular and cutaneous damage
  • pelvic fractures with severe bleeding, bladder and sciatic nerve damage.

132.
a. An old severely comminuted fracture–dislocation of the surgical neck of the upper humerus. Note the sclerosis showing that this fracture has been present for some time.
b. Injury to the circumflex (axillary) nerve and perhaps other neurological and vascular damage. The fracture may have been compound with secondary infection.
c. Extra-articular arthrodesis of the shoulder is probably the best treatment in a young male with about 60° abduction, 30° forward flexion and 30° internal rotation. In the elderly, a shoulder replacement should be considered if the circumflex nerve is intact. The post-operative X-rays shows a successful extra-articular arthrodesis by a posterior approach.

133.
a. Acute slip of the femoral capital epiphysis on the left side. In two thirds of cases it is a gradual process, whereas in one third the onset is sudden. Note the prominent lesser trochanter indicating that the leg is externally rotated.
b. Pain, limp, limited abduction and internal rotation, and increased external rotation. The leg externally rotates on flexion.

c. Pin in situ. Consider prophylactic pinning of the opposite hip. Both hips are affected in approximately 50% of cases. If the condition has been present for some time, an osteotomy to compensate for the slip can help.

134.
a. The X-ray shows a slightly displaced fracture of the acromion.
b. The fracture is recent as no callus formation is seen on the X-ray.
c. A triangular arm sling is worn for 1–2 weeks, followed by active exercises.

135.
a. Extensive burns. If burns cover more than 10% of the body, the patient must be admitted to hospital—especially in the case of children. Other indications for admission include all major full thickness burns and burns to the head, neck and perineum.
b. Fluid therapy in burns over 20% of body area (10% in children):
  • First 24 hours: crystalloid infusion of 20ml/kg/1st hour and measure urine output. If this is less than 0.5ml/kg/hour, increase drip rate. Blood transfusion and plasma infusion may also be necessary.
  • Second 24 hours: high-protein and albumin diet with oral fluids.
c. • Infection, toxaemia and renal failure.
  • Contractures and deformity.
  • Venous thrombosis and embolism.
  • Contracted joints—especially the hands.

136.
a. Olecranon bursitis—'student's elbow'. Other sites include prepatellar bursitis ('housemaid's knee') and infrapatellar bursitis ('clergyman's knee').
b. Constant friction and trauma.
c. Firm bandaging, avoid friction, give antiobiotics and drain if infected. Excise the bursa if necessary.

137.
a. The tear is usually caused by a twisting strain while weight bearing and therefore commonly seen in football and skiing.
b. The history may include a painful knee effusion, inability to fully straighten the leg, an unstable knee and a 'click' due to catching of the torn meniscus between the tibial plateau and the femoral condyle.
c. The medial collateral ligament attached to the meniscus may be damaged, as well as the anterior cruciate ligament.

138.
a. The common causes of this presentation include:
  • a complete tear of the supraspinatus tendon due to a

fall on to the shoulder plus age-related degeneration of the tendon due to osteoarthritis
- an incomplete tear of the supraspinatus tendon results in severe pain on attempted abduction of the shoulder.

Partial tears of the rotator cuff occur frequently with supraspinatus tendinitis due to avascular changes.

b. Only a small degree of abduction from a resting position is possible with scapular rotation. The deltoid muscle however cannot initiate further gleno-humeral abduction without the supraspinatus stabilising the joint first.

c. To distinguish between a partial and complete tear, a local anaesthetic can be injected below the acromion into the tendon to abolish pain. If the patient can now fully abduct the arm, the tear must only be partial.

139.
a. Spiral fracture of the right tibia and fibula.
b. Posterior tibial nerve.
c. Sensory loss over the sole of the foot with weakness of the intrinsic flexor muscles of the foot and toes.

140.
a. There is separation of the symphysis pubis (diastasis). On the left the pelvis is displaced superiorly. On the right there is a non-displaced fracture through the pubis and ischium.

b. Treatment options depending on the severity of the injury:
- Russell skin traction of 5 kg for 3–6 weeks
- Steinmann's pin inserted through the tibial tuberosity and 10–15 kg traction, reduced to 7 kg over 2–3 weeks and then maintained for 3–6 weeks
- external fixateur after reduction of the fracture (Fig. 140A) followed by plate fixation if necessary.

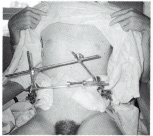

Fig 104A

c. The major early complication of this fracture is foot drop due to sciatic nerve damage. Other problems include: severe haemorrhage, damage to the bladder and urethra, backache and difficulty in sitting.

141.
a. Basic life support:
   - airway
   - breathing
   - circulation and blood loss.
b. This is an open, compound fracture, therefore:
   - vascular impairment of the toes
   - nerve defects
   - infection and osteomyelitis
   - other injuries elsewhere.

142. This man has an obvious left lower facial nerve palsy from injury to the nerve as it exits from the base of the skull. He is trying to close his eyes and show his teeth, but is unable to do so on the left side.

143.
a. Dislocated metacarpophalangeal joint of thumb—a hyperextension force dislocates the thumb backwards.
b. • Button hole deformity—it may need open reduction.
   - Associated fractures.
   - Instability with reduced pincer power.
   - Avulsion of tendon insertions.
   - Tearing of the joint capsule.
c. The metacarpophalangeal joint of the thumb is the most commonly dislocated joint in the hand, followed by the fifth finger.

144.
a. Fracture of the pubic rami and rupture of the membranous urethra with extravasation of urine into the extraperitoneal space, and displacement of the bladder superiorly.
b. Bleeding from the urethra. A rectal examination must never be omitted. It will demonstrate a gap anteriorly due to the upward displacement of the prostate. The patient will be in shock and may have other injuries requiring treatment.
c. Emergency repair and drainage of the bladder should be followed by insertion of suprapubic and urethral catheters after stabilisation of the patient's general condition. Most pubic fractures do not usually require treatment.

145.
a. The patient suffers from Pellegrini–Steida syndrome.
b. The condition arises from heterotopic ossification of the femoral origin of the medial collateral ligament. X-ray confirms the diagnosis. Considerable new bone may be formed due to tearing of the origin of the ligament, together with the adjacent periosteum. This causes localised bleeding with subsequent calcification and ossification which is made worse by repeated injury to an unstable knee.

146.
a. The X-ray demonstrates a stable, undisplaced spiral fracture of the 4th proximal phalanx. These fractures heal rapidly. Undisplaced fractures require little intervention. Initial splintage will reduce pain and maintain stability. After 2–3 weeks, active exercises should be commenced to avoid stiffness.

b. The main complication is malunion, especially if the fracture is unstable, and displacement occurs after reduction.

c. Fractures involving the articular surface are more difficult to treat and may progress to osteoarthritis. Fixation with K-wires may be necessary for displacement.

147.
a. Anterior dislocation of the shoulder with a fracture of the greater tuberosity with displacement.

b. The arm is held slightly abducted, flexed and internally rotated. The injury is usually due to forced abduction and external rotation of the arm due to a fall on the outstretched hand.

c. Complications of the injury include:
   • nerve injury (axillary nerve or brachial plexus) or vascular injury
   • fracture of the neck of the humerus
   • stiffness, pain and osteoarthritis
   • recurrent dislocation of the shoulder.
   Complications of reduction include fracture of the humerus, nerve and vascular injury.

148.
a. The X-ray shows a horizontal sclerotic area in the proximal tibia.

b. The patient has a healing stress fracture.

149.
a. There is a gap in the muscle belly of both quadriceps just proximal to the patellae due to rupture at their insertions. This injury usually occurs in the elderly due to forced flexion of the knee while actively extending.

b. Surgical repair is necessary to rejoin the muscle to the patella. Post-operative plaster immobilisation for 6 weeks should be followed by physiotherapy.

c. In young patients, rupture of the ligamentum patellae may occur following sporting injuries, while in middle age a transverse fracture of the patella is a complication of this type of injury.

150.
a. Posterior dislocation of the hip on the left, and anterior dislocation of the hip on the right. Note that the adducted, internally rotated hip is the posterior dislocation, and the

abducted externally rotated hip on the right is the anterior dislocation.
  b. Posterior dislocation can lead to damage to the sciatic nerve with a complete foot drop. It can also be associated with a fracture of the acetabulum which prevents stable reduction. Avascular necrosis of the head, with secondary osteoarthritis and myositis ossificans, are other complications.

151.
  a. Mothers with poor control of their diabetes in pregnancy give birth to large babies. In this case a difficult vaginal delivery led to trauma to the neonate.
  b. The X-ray shows a horizontal fracture of the upper third of the right femur with extensive callus formation.
  c. Fracture healing:
    1. Haematoma formation at and around the fracture site.
    2. Cells close to the periosteum proliferate.
    3. A cellular bridge forms in between the fracture ends.
    4. Callus forms consisting of osteophytes, osteoclasts, chondroblasts and fibroblasts.
    5. The immature bony bridge becomes mineralised.
    6. Woven early bone develops into stronger lamellar bone as the fracture consolidates.
    7. Remodelling with strengthening in the lines of stress.

152.
  a. Traumatic separation of C4 on C5 producing a high quadriplegia. There is an endotracheal tube in place.
  b. Poor. No spontaneous respiration as the lesion is at C4 and the diaphragm (C3,4,5) is paralysed. The child died within a week.

153.
Flexor tendon division is likely. This is a serious injury. Progressive adhesions in the flexor sheath may result in limited range of movement. Expert repair is necessary, often with tendon grafting. In addition, there may be digital nerve or vessel division.

154.
  a. No skin damage communicating with the fracture site.
  b. No—there may be significant blood loss into the musculature of the thigh (up to 1 to 2 litres).
  c. • Full views of joint above and below, i.e. of the hip and knee as associated fractures and dislocations of the hip and damage to the knee are common.
    • AP view of the pelvis.
    • Lateral X-ray of the femur.
    • X-ray any other sites of possible fracture or dislocation.

155.
  a. An ununited fracture of the shaft of the radius and ulna due to osteomyelitis. Sequestra, or regions of dead bone

surrounded by thickened new bone (involucrum), can be
seen adjacent to the fracture site. The chronic osteomyelitis
shown here is commonly seen after open fractures. It often
results in poor fracture healing with non-union.

b. Complications include vascular and neurological damage,
discharging sinuses, septicaemia, non-union and loss of
function of the forearm, particularly rotation.

c. Open fractures should be treated by excising sequestra
followed by intravenous antibiotics and a skin graft if
necessary. Later bone grafting may be necessary.

156.
a. Mid-tarsal dislocation.
b. Difficult to manage due to extensive pressure from oedema.
Requires immediate reduction to relieve pressure on the
neurovascular structures and especially the dorsalis pedis
artery which is often compressed. Kirschner wire fixation
followed by elevation and pressure dressing.
Immobilisation in a below-knee plaster splint when the
swelling has settled.

c. • Neurovascular compromise.
 • Associated fractures.
 • Infection.
 • Compartment syndrome of the foot with death of the
 intrinsic muscles of the foot and clawing of the toes.

157.
a. Transverse fracture of the shaft of humerus.
b. Radial nerve palsy.
c. Usually not. It can be placed in a good position and
maintained by non-operative means using a collar and
cuff sling. When the patient stands, the weight of the
arm applies traction across the fracture site. A plaster
U-slab provides more stability. Mobilisation is started
early.

158.
a. An old ununited fracture of the tibia and fibula with severe
angulation of the very thin bones. The pelvis shows an
increased valgus deformity of both necks of femur with
subluxation of the left hip.
b. Poliomyelitis with paralysis of both lower limbs.

159.
a. Posterior dislocation of elbow.
b. A fall onto the hand driving the forearm backwards.
c. Adequate muscle relaxant and anaesthesia must initially be
administered. The olecranon is pushed anteriorly while
the forearm is slowly flexed from the extended position.
Post-reduction X-ray is always necessary, as associated
fractures of the coronoid process of the ulna and head of
the radius are common. Post-operatively, the patient should

be splinted in an above elbow padded backslab or, alternatively, a collar and cuff sling for about 3 weeks.

160.
a. A Barton's fracture. The X-ray demonstrates a fracture line which runs into the wrist joint. The distal fragment is displaced anteriorly.
b. This fracture should be reduced in the same way as a Smith's fracture. A special T plate or Kirschner wire may be required.
c. Post-reduction, the fracture is easily redisplaced and inherently unstable. Other complications include:
  • stiffness of the fingers and wrist
  • malunion and instability
  • osteoarthritis of the wrist joint
  • rupture of the extensor pollicis longus tendon
  • Sudeck's atrophy with osteoporosis of the wrist bones due to autonomic involvement
  • median and occasionally ulnar nerve compression.

161.
a. The X-ray shows malunion or an old hypertrophic non-union of a fractured shaft of humerus. Other X-rays and a tomogram, nuclear bone scan or a CT scan may be necessary if clinical examination is equivocal.
b. The deformity can be corrected by excising the sclerotic bone ends or stabilising the fracture with a locking nail or plate plus bone graft. This is a difficult operation as the radial nerve is often adherent to the fracture. In this patient the mobile painless pseudoarthrosis was left untreated.
c. Delayed union may be caused by:
  • infection
  • markedly displaced bone ends with interposed muscle
  • excessive movement at the fracture site
  • inadequate blood supply
  • pathological bone including secondary deposits and Paget's disease.

162.
a. Bullet wounds to his spine.
b. Paraplegia with sensory, motor and autonomic involvement with bed sores, contractures and bladder paralysis. He may also have penetration into his abdomen with injury to the spleen, liver, kidneys, intestines and other abdominal organs.

163.
a. Dislocated patella (Fig. 163A).
b. Closed reduction, immobilise with splint for 6 weeks.
c. • Patella alta (high-riding patella)

- Undeveloped lateral femoral condyle
- Genu valgum, particularly in overweight adolescent girls.

164.
a. The zygoma has probably been fractured.
b. A direct injury as this bone forms the prominence of the cheek.
c. Depressed fractures, which if not treated promptly may lead to a flat cheek which will prove difficult to reconstruct later. Infraorbital anaesthesia is a common disturbing symptom which may take many years to recover.

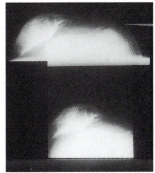
Fig 163A

165.
a. Varus deformity of the lower left tibia due to malunion, with gross shortening of the lower leg. There is a surgical scar over the anterior surface of the tibia. The leg has been shaved prior to surgery. This fracture is the result of a motorcycle accident.
b. Operative correction with osteotomy and internal fixation with an electrical bone stimulator or bone graft, or both. Post-operative physiotherapy for stiff ankle and a raised shoe for shortening of the leg.
c. The altered biomechanics of the knee and ankle joint, due to the angulation, may lead to osteoarthritis of these joints.

166.
a. Supracondylar fracture of humerus.
b. • Brachial artery injury (occlusion or division).
   • Flexor compartment syndrome with Volkmann's ischaemic contracture of the flexor forearm muscles.
   • Radial or anterior interosseous, and median and ulnar nerve lesions.
   • Elbow stiffness, mainly loss of extension.
   • Malunion or epiphyseal damage with cubitus varus or valgus.
c. Supracondylar fractures are very common in children.

167.
a. Acromioclavicular complete dislocation.
b. Fall onto the point of the shoulder.
c. Triangular sling for 3 weeks and early mobilisation. Occasionally internal fixation is required, usually in young women and mainly for cosmesis.

168.
a. The radial nerve causing a wrist drop.
b. Lesions at several common sites produce this picture:
   - High lesions—due to trauma or pressure to the axilla, e.g. with crutches. The triceps muscle is also compromised.
   - Humeral lesions—due to fractures to the shaft of the humerus.
   - Low lesions—due to fracture/dislocations at the elbow.
c. The sensory loss is over the dorsal aspect of the hand at the base of the 1st and 2nd fingers, extending to the wrist.

169.
a. There is an incomplete greenstick fracture of the base of the neck of femur. In a child, part of the periosteum in this type of fracture remains in continuity. Do *not* confuse this with *normal* epiphysis seen in this X-ray.
b. • Bed rest and skin traction.
   • Hip spica, crutches and early mobility.

170.
a. The X-ray shows avascular necrosis of the proximal pole of the scaphoid following a fracture of the waist of the scaphoid.
b. Severe osteoarthritis with a destroyed wrist joint.

171.
a. The patient had an established non-union of a subtrochanteric femoral fracture.
b. This is a poor area for healing due to damage to the nutrient artery. He was using two of the broken nails as fishing sinkers (see p. 87). He was unwilling to give these up unless success was assured with treatment.
c. The treatment of choice is a Huckstep titanium locking nail with bone graft and elongation by 4 cm (Fig. 171A). It is essential to bone graft the defect (as in this case) from cancellous bone taken from the patient's iliac crest. Union occurred in 4 months.

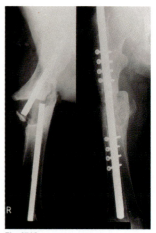

Fig 171A

172.
a. Ulnar nerve palsy demonstrating an 'ulnar claw hand'.
b. Froment's sign—the loss of thumb adduction by the ulnar nerve is compensated for by exaggerated interphalangeal

flexion by flexor pollicis longus (innervated by the median nerve) during strong pinch. The hand will also have weak interosseous function—abduction and adduction of the fingers plus extension of the 4th and 5th fingers at the interphalangeal joints as shown in the photo.

c. Sensory loss may include the medial third of the palm, half the fourth finger and the whole fifth digit.

173.

a. A seat belt injury. Note the diagonal bruising from the left shoulder to the right abdomen. This was due to a non-retractable seat belt that was too loose.

b. Possible complications of this are a fractured clavicle, fractured ribs with penetration of the lung and a tension pneumothorax and haemothorax, damage to the pericardium with a haemopericardium and cardiac tamponade, and possible damage to the liver. The patient also had a head and cervical and thoracic spinal injuries. She could also have sustained injuries to other abdominal organs, including the ascending colon, pancreas and small intestine. She may also have injuries to the lumbar spine, pelvis and limbs.

174.

a. 'MAST'—Military Anti-Shock Trousers. These are pneumatic compression trousers used as a temporary emergency measure to splint fractures of the lower limb and pelvis, and to prevent pooling of blood in the lower limbs in the case of severe blood loss. One to two litres of blood can be prevented from pooling.

b. • The three compartments of the trousers must all be inflated by mouth or by a hand pump with a pressure limiter.
  • These should only be deflated gradually once intravenous fluid and blood replacement has been given and the patient's condition has been stabilised.
  • Care should be taken with transport by air or land over 1000 metres, or when putting the patient in the hot sun; under these conditions the pressure in the trousers can increase resulting in ischaemia and gangrene of the feet if left for more than six hours.

175.

a. The 'Boxer's fracture', although it tends to be the bar-room brawler. The true pugilist hits with his 2nd and 3rd metacarpals. A fracture may occur to the neck of one of these, as well as to either the trapezoid and capitate bones of the wrist.

b. Splintage is unnecessary apart from an aluminium cock-up

splint for a few days. The patient is encouraged to mobilise early.

c. A loss of prominence of the 5th knuckle is common, but does not compromise hand function. Osteoarthritis of the metacarpophalangeal joints is a common complication of boxing.

176.
a. Indications include:
- peripheral vascular disease—due to atherosclerosis
- severe trauma, e.g. motor vehicle and industrial accidents
- primary tumours of bone or soft tissue
- malformations, either congenital or acquired
- severe nerve damage, i.e. brachial plexus injury.

b. Early complications include infection and gas gangrene. The skin flaps may 'break down' due to excessive tension on the wound. In severe peripheral vascular disease, the stump may become ischaemic and re-amputation may be necessary.

c. Yes! 'Phantom limb pain' is a pathological phenomenon giving the patient the feeling that the limb is still present. It is minimised by coagulation diathermy to all nerves before division at the time of amputation.

177.
The apparently raised diaphragm is actually a ruptured diaphragm with intestine in the chest.

178.
a. Complications include:
- bronchopneumonia
- pressure areas with ulcers over the heel, greater trochanters and sacrum
- flexion contractures of the hips and knees
- deep venous thrombosis and pulmonary embolus
- urinary tract infection with cystitis, ascending pyelitis nephritis and death
- mental disorientation.

b. Immediate operative fixation of the fracture with early mobilisation out of bed the following day and early full weight bearing.

179.
a. Stable lumbar vertebral fracture of L2 where there is loss of vertebral height to less than 50%.

b. Conservative treatment is required with:
- bed rest with the mattress on fracture boards for 3 days to 3 weeks
- analgesics
- back support and local heat
- education—to avoid back strain.

The latter includes a pillow in the middle of the back when sitting, lifting with a straight back, a lumbosacral support and back exercises at home. Swimming is the ideal exercise for patients with back problems.

180.
a. The photograph shows a flap of skin which has been sheared off, probably due to a blunt injury. The wound appears to involve the muscle and fascial layers. ·
b. The damaged structures include:
  • extensor tendon to the middle finger
  • digital nerves and vessels
  • fractures of the metacarpals and phalanges
  • muscle and skin.
c. Examinations should include:
  • extension at the interphalangeal joints
  • test for sensation over the middle finger
  • assess vascular insufficiency, by sensation, coldness and capillary return
  • X-ray the part for bony injury and foreign bodies.
Finally, explore and debride the wound under anaesthesia.

181.
a. Mallet finger.
b. Simple splint in hyperextension of the distal interphalangeal joint for 6 weeks (Fig. 181A).
c. Rupture of the extensor tendon of the terminal phalanx or avulsion of bone at the tendon insertion.

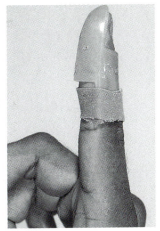
Fig 181A

182.
a. Haemarthrosis due to a fracture into the knee joint. The diagnosis is made from the fat globules in the kidney dish, which indicate a fracture of the adjacent bones to the joint. A fracture must be looked for carefully when fat globules are seen.
b. A haemarthrosis without fat globules may occur with any major partial or complete ligamentous rupture, without a fracture. A synovial effusion with straw-coloured fluid occurs following injuries to the meniscus, minor injuries to the ligaments and in osteoarthritis and rheumatoid arthritis. Extensive bleeding usually occurs immediately after injury, often more than 50 ml, while a synovial effusion may take

several hours to develop, and is often less than 50 ml. An infected arthritis will result in a cloudy fluid or frank pus, depending on the organism.

183.
a. An undisplaced avulsion fracture of the greater tuberosity of the humerus.
b. A fall onto the shoulder is usually responsible. The supraspinatus tendon attaches here, and may pull the fragment away from its attachment. This may prevent full abduction of the shoulder due to impingement on the acromion.
c. Older patients are mainly affected. Shoulder dislocation in a younger patient may, however, have an associated fracture.
d. The fragment usually unites in a satisfactory position. A triangular sling and physiotherapy is the usual treatment. Displaced fragments will require open reduction and internal fixation.

184.
a. Trochanteric fracture of the upper femur. These fractures are usually comminuted.
b. There may be considerable blood loss into the surrounding tissues with swelling of the lateral side of the upper thigh.
c. The leg is usually externally rotated 90° with bruising over the fracture site.

185.
a. The right arm is held in extension and internal rotation—the 'waiter's tip' position.
b. Paralysis of the C5 and C6 nerve roots due to birth trauma, especially in breech deliveries. The shoulder abductors, external rotators and the biceps are paralysed. Sensation is lost along the outer aspect of the arm.
c. Erb's palsy.
d. The majority of cases recover without treatment.

186. A severe compound infected fracture of the ulna with loss of most of the shaft due to previous injury and infection. Note the protrusion of the head of the radius into the lower humerus, the false elbow joint and the new bone formation showing that this injury probably occurred several years previously.

187.
a. The medial collateral ligament (MCL) has been ruptured, from either a direct valgus force applied to the knee or external rotation of the tibia, or both. The lateral plateau of the tibia or lateral femoral condyle could also be fractured.
b. Third degree severe tears may result in an 'unhappy triad' of injuries:
   • Medial collateral ligament injury. The medial meniscus

is attached to the medial ligament and is detached in severe injuries.
- Anterior cruciate ligament rupture.
- Lateral meniscal injury as the medial compartment opens up and compresses the lateral compartment.

188.
a. Anterior dislocation of the right hip. The leg is externally rotated, abducted and flexed. An X-ray must be taken to exclude an associated fracture of the anterior rim of the acetabulum or a fracture of the neck of the femur. A CT scan may also be necessary after the hip has been reduced.
b. Reduction is achieved with the aid of a relaxant anaesthetic. Manipulation with flexion of the hip and internal rotation and adduction of the leg.
c. Anterior dislocation is very uncommon compared to posterior dislocation. The most important acute complication is damage to the femoral vessels and nerve.

189.
a. This X-ray taken in casualty shows a completely displaced, oblique fracture of the tibia and fibula with subsequent disruption of the ankle joint stability—a so called 'third degree' fracture/dislocation of the ankle.
b. This fracture will require internal reduction and fixation to minimise complications and to restore stability to the joint.
c. Complications include:
   - vascular and neurological damage
   - damage to skin with osteomyelitis or pyogenic arthritis
   - non-union or malunion
   - late osteoarthritis of the ankle
   - instability
   - stiffness and pain.

190.
a. The young boy has an ununited fracture of the clavicle due to a fracture about 2 years previously as an infant.
b. This shows the typical 'tenting' over his clavicle caused by the growth of the bone.

191.
a. 'Popeye's' arm—from traumatic rupture of the long head of the tendon of biceps. It is a tear through an area of avascular degeneration in the bicipital groove and is usually associated with degenerative arthritis of the shoulder.
b. In the acute rupture, surgical repair is possible but not usually necessary. If left alone, the patient's discomfort soon disappears and good function returns without further treatment.

192.
a. There is dislocation of the proximal interphalangeal joint of the middle finger. This is a very common injury, especially in young patients involved with ball sports.

b. An X-ray both before and after reduction is essential to exclude associated fractures and to check the adequacy of the reduction. Collateral ligaments are sometimes damaged and should be tested by gentle lateral stressing. If a ligament is torn, surgical repair may sometimes be necessary. The finger should be splinted on a metal splint, in slight flexion for several days.

193.
a. A severely angulated fracture of the mid shaft of the humerus which has been badly treated with a large plaster cast which is causing the large opaque shadow around the humerus.

194.
'A E I O U—Cardiovascular system—Don't Forget Them'
A lcohol
E pilepsy
I njury including electrical accidents
O piates and other drugs
U raemia and metabolic disturbances
C ardiovascular system—cardiac, cerebrovascular (i.e. stroke), shock etc.
D iabetes: hypoglycaemic and hyperglycaemic
F unctional and fat embolus
T hermal (heat stroke) and tropical (i.e. malaria).

195.
Intra-articular dislocation of patella—an exceedingly rare injury where the patella has been avulsed from quadriceps tendon.

196.
a. Bennett's fracture dislocation of the carpometacarpal joint.
b. Traction on the thumb with adduction of the metacarpal and pressure over the base of the metacarpal. The fracture will usually reduce easily. Achieving reduction is easy, but maintaining it is more difficult in a scaphoid type plaster for 6 weeks with the thumb adducted. Percutaneous K-wires, or screw fixation may be necessary.
c. A sesamoid bone in the short flexor tendon.

197.
a. A fracture of the shaft of a metacarpal. The diagnosis is suspected by the appearance of the tender and swollen hand.
b. Stable, as it is splinted by adjacent interosseous muscles and other metacarpals.
c. Supportive bandage or aluminium cock-up splint for several days and early mobilisation.

198.
a. There is a small medial fracture of the margin of the patella on this 'skyline' view.
b. This is probably due to a recurrent dislocation of the patella.
c. A bipartite patella which is a congenital deformity. This is

usually not tender and may be bilateral. It has a sharp edge signifying that it has been present for a long time.

199.
a. The X-ray shows a depressed fracture of the skull, commonly following an injury with a small hard object. Child abuse should be excluded. The anterior fontanelle has not closed so the patient is under 18 months of age.
b. The dura is usually torn.
c. Following severe head trauma, investigations such as cervical and skull X-rays should be carried out. Neurological monitoring using the Glasgow coma scale is necessary while awaiting expert neurosurgical advice. Definitive treatment in this case includes disimpaction of the fracture and evacuation of any subdural haematoma.

200.
a. This is the anterior drawer test where the patient's foot is immobilised under the examiner's thigh, and the tibia drawn forward on the lower femur.
b. A positive test is shown where there is anterior displacement of the tibia on the femur from rupture of the anterior cruciate ligament.
c. The anterior cruciate ligament is best repaired arthroscopically in young active patients. Older patients often manage well with occasional brace use and physiotherapy.

201.
a. This is an old fracture since there is callus formation, resorption of bone ends and osteoporosis around the fracture site.
b. Clinical signs of bony union include an absence of movement and tenderness at the fracture site, especially on stressing the fracture.

202.
a. A large cyst with sclerotic margins in the lunate with avascular changes. He also has a recent fracture of the lower end of the radius and evidence of osteoarthritis of the wrist.
b. An old dislocated lunate and a recent fracture of the radius.

203.
a. This X-ray shows a non-displaced vertical split fracture of the lateral tibial plateau.
b. This injury is usually caused by the lateral condyle of the femur exerting excessive force on the lateral plateau of the tibia. A tear of the medial

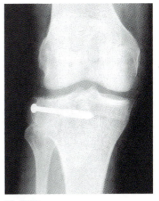

Fig 203A

collateral ligament may be associated. Direct trauma to the lateral aspect of the knee, from the bumper of a car is a common cause.

c. Immediate treatment on arrival at a casualty department includes joint aspiration of the haemarthrosis and examination for soft tissue (e.g. medial ligament), neurological or vascular damage. An AP and lateral X-ray of the knee should be carried out. An oblique X-ray or a CT scan may also be necessary to show depression of the lateral plateau of the tibia. Internal fixation (Fig. 203A, p. 152) and early mobilisation of the knee in displaced fractures will usually be necessary.

204.

a. • Splenic, liver and renal damage.
   • Penetration of the stomach, colon and small intestine.
   • Neurovascular damage.

b. Emergency priorities:
   • resuscitate patient
   • place in two large bore intravenous cannulas for volume replacement
   • take blood for group, cross match and hold
   • organise a theatre for an emergency laparotomy.

205.

a. There are multiple abrasions on the left side of his face. On closer inspection there is meiosis and ptosis of the left eye.

b. Horner's syndrome—due to a traumatic injury to the sympathetic chain. This could be secondary to the lateral flexion of the head from the shoulder associated with a fall from a height.

c. It will feel dry—anhydrosis. Remember 'MAPE':
   M eiosis—constricted pupil.
   A nhydrosis—lack of sweating and a dry forehead.
   P tosis—a 'dropped' eyelid.
   E nopthalmos—the eye ball sunken into the orbit.

206.

a. Fractured right neck of femur with associated secondary osteoporosis is commonly seen in females over 60.

b. Postmenopausal osteoporosis. Hormone replacement therapy (oestrogens) in these patients may slow down or even stop the osteoporosis. They should also be encouraged to take daily exercises and a balanced diet high in calcium plus vitamin D to help the absorption of calcium after external fixation of the fracture.

c. Bone density studies—these tests are indicated in patients with osteoporosis or a metabolic bone disease with a resultant loss of bone mass. The test provides a 'fracture risk' for these patients.

Further reading list

Adams, J.C., Hamblen D.L. *Outline of Fractures* Churchill Livingstone, Edinburgh

Adams, J.C., Hamblen D.L. *Outline of Orthopaedics* Churchill Livingstone, Edinburgh

Apley, A.G., Solomon, L. *Concise System of Orthopaedics and Fractures* Butterworths, London

Apley, A.G., Solomon, L. *Apley's System of Orthopaedics and Fractures* Butterworth, London

Dandy, D.J. *Essential Orthopaedics and Trauma* Churchill Livingstone, Edinburgh

Hooper, G. *Orthopaedics (Colour Guide)* Churchill Livingstone, Edinburgh

Huckstep, R.L. *A Simple Guide to Trauma* Churchill Livingstone, Edinburgh

Huckstep, R.L. *A Simple Guide to Orthopaedics* Churchill Livingstone, Edinburgh

Index

Note: entries are indexed **by question** numbers and matching answers.